PSYCHIATRY- THEORY, APPLICATIONS, AND TREATMENTS SERIES



# STRESS OF FAMILY MEMBERS IN CARING FOR A RELATIVE WITH SCHIZOPHRENIA

# PSYCHIATRY- THEORY, APPLICATIONS, AND TREATMENTS SERIES

**Attention Deficit Hyperactivity Disorder (ADHD)**
*Stuart M. Gordon and Aileen E. Mitchell (Editors)*
2009 ISBN: 978-1-60741-581-7

**Attention Deficit Hyperactivity Disorder (ADHD)**
*Stuart M. Gordon and Aileen E. Mitchell (Editors)*
2009. ISBN: 978-1-60876-699-4 (Online Book)

**War and Suicide**
*Leo Sher and Alexander Vilens (Editors)*
2009. ISBN: 978-1-60741-978-5

**Dyslexia and Depression: The Hidden Sorrow**
*Neil Alexander-Passe*
2010. ISBN: 978-1-60876-118-0

**Stress of Family Members in Caring for a Relative with Schizophrenia**
*Wai-Tong Chien*
2010. ISBN: 978-1-60876-145-6

PSYCHIATRY- THEORY, APPLICATIONS, AND TREATMENTS SERIES

# STRESS OF FAMILY MEMBERS IN CARING FOR A RELATIVE WITH SCHIZOPHRENIA

WAI-TONG CHIEN

**Nova Science Publishers, Inc.**
*New York*

For permission to use material from this book please contact us:
Telephone 631-231-7269; Fax 631-231-8175
Web Site: http://www.novapublishers.com



LIBRARY OF CONGRESS CATALOGING-IN-PUBLICATION DATA

ISBN: 978-1-60876-145-6

Available upon request.

*Published by Nova Science Publishers, Inc. ✦ New York*

# CONTENTS

# PREFACE

The number of people with schizophrenia globally is estimated at about 35 million, of whom 20 million live in developing or less developed countries. Despite the rapid development in pharmacological and psychosocial treatment of schizophrenia, the dissemination of psychosocial interventions as usual practice within mental health services has been slow and patchy. Specialized care and psychoscial interventions may be a means of engaging patients in community mental health services and reducing patients' relapse from illness; however, limited evidence exists because of wide variations in implementation with little guidance or inadequate funding from the health authorities towards early detection, community-based intervention, and outpatient care services to prevent relapse. Many newly-invented neuroleptic drugs can give patients partial protection against environmental stress, but they need to be supplemented with a therapeutic social environment, especially a healthy and supportive family. Families, particularly those members who live with a relative with schizophrenia often face daily stressors which include the patient's unpredictable and bizarre behaviors, the external stressors of social stigma and isolation, emotional frustration such as guilt and loneliness, and family conflicts which arise during the caring process. Nevertheless, these families are inadequately prepared and supported for such caregiving tasks and demands. Thus, this book also addresses an important question of family care: "Are family interventions effective in promoting health and other benefits for families of people with schizophrenia?"

# ABSTRACT

A review was undertaken to assess the relative effectiveness of different modes of family intervention for family caregivers of people suffering from schizophrenia. A literature search was undertaken to fill in gaps in the knowledge of the psychological distress and burden encountered by these family caregivers and whether family intervention (involving different kinds of psychosocial interventions for family caregivers) can help these caregivers improve their caregiving and psychological well-being. A broad range of electronic bibliographic databases in medicine, health care, nursing, psychology and social sciences (e.g., Cochrane Database of Systematic Reviews, Embase, Medline, DARE, Ovid, PsycINFO, and Social Sciences Citation Index) were searched from 1985 to 2008, and the searches were restricted to English language. The results highlight the increasing attention given to family caregivers' distress and burden among these mentally ill clients, as well as the number of research studies and controlled trials of family intervention. The findings of these studies have established a more sound evidence base on the effect of family environment, particularly those inducing life stressors and burden, on both mentally ill clients and their family members. Family-focused intervention for these clients should be carefully designed and implemented to meet their health needs.

# INTRODUCTION

According to the World Health Organization (2007), the number of people with schizophrenia globally is estimated at about 35 million, 20 million of whom live in developing or less developed countries. Despite the rapid development in pharmacological and psychosocial treatment of schizophrenia, the common practice of dissemination of psychosocial interventions within mental health services has been slow and patchy (Barbato & D'Avanzo, 2000; Penn & Mueser, 1996). Specialized care and new early intervention services may be a means of engaging patients in community mental health services and reducing patients' re-hospitalizations; however, limited evidence exists because of wide variations in implementation with little guidance or inadequate funding from the health authorities towards early detection, home treatment, and services to prevent relapse (Craig et al., 2004). Many newly-invented neuroleptic drugs can give patients partial protection against environmental stress, but they need to be supplemented with a therapeutic social environment, especially a healthy and supportive family. However, the shortcomings of community care have produced many negative consequences for both the families and their mentally ill relatives, who are often coerced into the service to compensate for the deficiencies of the community care system (Chien et al., 2005; Saunders, 1999).

In Western and Asian countries, it has been estimated that more than 70% of schizophrenic patients discharged from hospitals live with family members or stay in regular contact with them and depend on their care (Chan & Yu, 2004; Heller, Roccoforte & Cook, 1997). Families, particularly those family members who live with their schizophrenic relative, often face daily stressors including the patient's unpredictable and bizarre behavior, external stressors of social stigma and isolation, emotional frustration such as guilt and loneliness, and family conflicts that arise during the caring process (Leff, 1994). Studies have shown that family caregivers may report psychological distress, social and family disharmony, and practical problems in living with and taking care of the patient at home. Similarly, Brooker (2001) and Canive et al. (1996) describe family caregivers as suffering from depression, anxiety, grief and somatic complaints, as well as disruption to their social and leisure activities and domestic routine and reduction in household income. Therefore, caregiving for family members with schizophrenia is extremely stressful and burdensome, with negative consequences for the social and psychological health of the caregivers, indicating the importance of health professionals in providing family-oriented mental health care (Loukissa, 1995).

The impact of caring for persons with schizophrenia and other severe mental illnesses is often described as burdensome and includes the physical, psychological or emotional, social, and financial problems experienced by family caregivers, representing both subjective and objective aspects of the impact of care (Marsh, 1998). Research from the mid 1950s (Clausen & Yarrow, 1955) has indicated that the caregivers' psychological well-being can be seriously impaired and, subsequently, family burden has become an increasingly important area of concern in studies on family caregiving.

Due to the importance of the bio-psychosocial impacts of caring for schizophrenic persons on family members, there is a need to understand the concepts of stress/distress and caregiving burden among the family caregivers of clients with schizophrenia. In addition, a number of literature reviews that examined the effects of family interventions on people with schizophrenia have either focused primarily on a few approaches of intervention frequently used and empirically tested in mental health research, such as psycho-education programs (Dixon, Adams and Luckstead, 2000), or examined only randomized controlled trials (Pharoah et al., 2001). There is a notable omission of alternative approaches to family intervention, such as cognitive behavioral technique, behavioral management programs and mutual support groups. Given the increasing emphasis of self-help programs and family-based interventions in mental health services in the United States (U.S.), the United Kingdom (U.K.), and other developed Western countries, mutual support groups would be considered one of the potential alternatives to family intervention for schizophrenia. The aim of this literature review was to establish what is known about the concepts of caregiving stress and burden, and the relative effectiveness of different common approaches of family intervention for people suffering from schizophrenia. Thus, this review also addresses an important question of family care: "Are family interventions effective in promoting health and other benefits for families of people with schizophrenia?"

*Chapter 1*

# LITERATURE SEARCH STRATEGY

This review of the research literature was based on the procedures suggested by the National Health Service Centre for Reviews and Dissemination (2001) Report Number 4 in the U.K. Databases searched were Medline, Embase, CINAHL, OVID full text, PsycINFO, the Cochrane Library, the NHS National Research Register, and System for Info on Grey Literature. The *British Journal of Psychiatry*, the *Schizophrenia Bulletin*, *American Journal of Psychiatry* and other psychiatry and psychology journals available at the university libraries (i.e., both English and Chinese languages) were hand-searched, and reference lists of all retrieved literature were also searched to identify studies that may have been missed. Leading researchers of current studies, as identified on the National Research Register, were contacted to ascertain if a research report or paper relating to this intervention was due for publication during this review.

A combined free-text and thesaurus approach was adopted to search electronic databases. "Population" search terms included severe mental illness, psychos*, and schizophreni*. "Intervention" search terms included family intervention, psychoeducat*, individual or group therap*, family therap*, family work, and mutual support or self help. "Concept" search terms included stress, distress, caregiver or caregiving burden, family members, carer or caregivers, and coping. The search strategy was restricted to English-language research articles published from 1988 to 2008, except for those imposed by the databases themselves.

For the literature on family intervention, two inclusion criteria were used to guide the search strategy: (a) the intervention used should be a family or professional-led program for families of a relative with schizophrenia or other psychotic disorder; and (b) only quantitative research was selected. Systematic review and meta-analysis of this topic were also searched. A total of 637 articles were retrieved from the electronic databases, of which one-fifth (n=120) were found to be relevant and appropriate for further review. Hand searching, tracing unpublished or in-press research reports, and screening reference lists increased the total number of articles retrieved for critical review to 140. After an examination for relevance of these retrieved articles on family intervention in schizophrenia, 100 were excluded, mainly because they were brief reports, discussion papers, qualitative studies, or publications repeating the findings of the same study. Finally, a total of 40 studies were reviewed for this chapter, consisting of 16 studies using an experimental or randomized controlled trial design; 10 using a quasi-experimental design (non-equivalent comparison groups); three using a longitudinal non-equivalent group design (two time points at one-year interval); five using a cross-sectional comparative group survey design (participants vs. non-participants); three using a single cohort pre-test and post-test design; and three using a cross-sectional descriptive survey design.

For the literature on the concepts of burden and stress, a total of 113 articles were retrieved from both the electronic database and hand searching, of which 38 were found to be relevant and appropriate for further review. After examination for clarity and comprehensiveness of these retrieved articles, 18 were accepted for review in the chapter, consisting of five full research reports and 10 theoretical or discussion papers and three editorial and commentary papers.

*Chapter 2*

# STRESS IN FAMILY CAREGIVING

The basic assumption and philosophy of the treatment model of severe mental illness is more acceptable when mental illness can be viewed under the stress-vulnerability model (Kuipers, Leff & Lam, 2002). Kuipers et al. describes this model as a bio-psychosocial approach, in which at times of extremely stressful situations—for example, solitary confinement, sleep deprivation and acute physical illness—transient psychotic symptoms can be manifested in any person. It appears that such a stress model can also be applied to family caregivers of these mentally ill individuals. Stressors in caregiving may combine the impacts of the patients' psychotic symptoms, and problem behaviors with the other negative life factors encountered by individual family members or the entire family as a whole, to place the family system under strain. Even though the model has been used to explain a wide range of responses to stressors induced by acute or chronic mental illness, there is limited research on its application to family caregiving, with the exception of a few studies on dementia care (Schultz & Beach, 1999).

However, the stress-vulnerability model also argues that certain characteristics or experiences make some people more vulnerable to stress. Stressful events are not additive, but interact with the characteristics or experiences of individuals to increase distress more rapidly among people in the "vulnerable" group (Schultz & Sherwood, 2008). As with the vulnerability, the levels of strains (ambient stress) can vary from person to person. Family members who find the illness difficult to accept or adjust to can become critical of the ill relative, as they are unaware of the effects of the illness or extremely frustrated with the challenges they have to deal with (Brennan, 2000). They can also over-compensate for the illness and can infringe the ill relative's autonomy in an attempt to ensure that the relative is cared for. Such so-called "high expressed emotion" families or caregivers can unwittingly increase the level of everyday ambient stress for individual caregivers as well as for the ill relative (Leff & Vaughn, 1985).

Expressed emotion (EE) refers to the degree of criticism, hostility and emotional involvement in family relationships and interactions with a mentally ill patient (Gerlsma & Hale III, 1997; Vaughn & Leff, 1976). Although many studies have supported the hypothesis that high EE is one important family attribute in the etiology of schizophrenia, recent studies have failed to confirm this (Raune, Kuipers & Bebbington, 2004; Wearden et al., 2000). Indeed, there is a growing body of evidence to support the assertion that family members' beliefs about schizophrenia, their appraisals of the stress in caregiving and the patient's level of control over their own symptoms are associated with the level of EE (Raune et al., 2004). Wearden et al. (2000) have argued that if family caregivers considered patients' symptoms to be controllable and internal, they would attempt to coerce the patient to get back to normal (higher EE in terms of criticism and hostility) as their coping response. Barrowclough et al. (2001) and Scazufca and Kuipers (1999) have acknowledged that EE may represent the complex interactions between patients and family caregivers and, indeed, the patients' illness and behaviors are an important part of the process contributing to the origins and changes in EE within a family over time. In Western countries, EE has also been proved to be a more generalized risk factor for relapse in different mental health problems such as schizophrenia, depression, dementia, and anxiety disorders (Gerlsma & Hale III, 1997; Wearden et al., 2000). Studies have also indicated that the level of EE correlates closely with patients' adherence to medications (Flanagan & Wagner, 1991; Wearden et al., 2000), their level of functioning, and their likelihood of psychiatric relapse (Butzlaff & Hooley, 1998).

Kuipers et al. (2002), therefore, suggest that instead of families being blamed for the mental illness, they are encouraged to be therapeutic agents in order to help their mentally ill member. They have strengths of love, intimacy and long-lasting family relationships with the ill relative, which cannot be replaced by somebody else. On the other hand, families are seen as bearing high levels of physical and psychological strains in the long process of caregiving and, thus, are overwhelmed by the distress and burden of caring for their family members with psychosis—a factor that is taken very seriously.

Mental health effects of caregiving may include depression, anxiety, sense of burden, and reduced quality of life and self-efficacy in life situations (Schultz & Beach, 1999). A greater degree of depression and stress and low ratings of subjective quality of life in caregiving are consistently and positively associated with a number of factors, including the mentally ill relative's behavior problems and functional disabilities; duration and amount of care provided; the caregiver's age; and the relationship between caregiver and the ill relative (Vitaliano, Zhang & Scanlan, 2003). Recently, researchers have also found that a caregiver's perception of the degree to which the ill relative is suffering is a major cause of distress (Nolan, Lundh, Grant & Keady, 2003). Nevertheless, the physical effects of caregiving, such as sleep deprivation and exhaustion, are generally less intensive than the psychological effects, regardless of whether they are assessed by global self-report scales or physiologic measures such as stress hormone levels (Brown, Birley & Wing, 1972; Fadden, 2001). Although relatively few studies have focused on the relationships between family caregiving and the health habits of caregivers, researchers have found evidence of impaired health behaviors, such as neglecting their own health care management or medical follow-up and eating poor-quality foods, among some caregivers (Schultz & Sherwood, 2008).

*Chapter 3*

# Concept of Family Burden

Family, caregiver or caregiving burden are terms frequently used to refer to the totality of the experience of caring for an ill relative, including effects on the physical, psychological and socio-economic well-being, as well as the capacity to cope with and adjust to that circumstance (Rose, Mallinson & Walton-Moss, 2002). From the 1970s to the 1980s, the adverse consequences of mental illness for family caregivers, known as family burden, have been studied to either determine the feasibility of discharging a patient into their community or to refine the concept of caregiving and its underlying structure and content (Schene, Tessler & Gamache, 1994). Since then, the concept of family burden has become universal—with numerous studies in the West and relatively fewer works from the Eastern world, e.g., Asia and Australia (Ustun, 1999)—and there have been at least 17 reviews of caregiving experience and burden for patients with severe mental illness from 1987 to 2002 (Ohaeri, 2003). Studies have indicated consistently that there may be severe distress and burden upon the whole family in living with a relative with schizophrenia, particularly for the primary caregiver, because family members' needs are often superseded by those of the patient (Maurin & Boyd, 1990). The U.S. administration proposed a $6 billion five-year project to address the long-term care needs of patients with chronic mental illness and their families (Arno, Levine & Memmott, 1999), whereas in the U.K., the National Service Framework for Mental Health reported by the Department of Health (1999) recommended that caregivers' health needs such as psychological distress and caregiving burden should be taken into account when providing community-based care to patients with severe mental illness in the U.K. (Treasure et al., 2001).

In recent years, the concept of burden has been broadened into a multi-dimensional construct (Woods, Haberman & Packard, 1993). Using rating scales, the concept of family burden is quantified as objective burden, which refers to the observable consequences of caregiving on family life such as financial loss, impairment of work efficiency, and disruption of family routines; and subjective burden, which refers to the psychological reactions and attitudes towards caregiving, such as attitudes toward the patient, emotional climate at home, and subjective feeling of difficulty coping with the illness when these problems are attributable to the illness (Schene, 1990). As the concept of caregiver burden has become more specific and widely used in family caregiving research (Dunkin & Hanley, 1998), different aspects of caregiving burden experienced by family members—including physical, psychological, social, and financial problems—are emphasized and studied using a standardized instrument such as the Family Burden Interview Schedule used in this study (Chou, 2000; Schene, Tessler & Gamanche, 1994). This is an important outcome measure in intervention studies for family caregivers of patients with chronic and mental illnesses (Chien & Norman, 2004).

Because individual caregivers respond differently to the stressors of caregiving situations, researchers have identified factors that affect the relationship between the demands of care and the caregiver burden and distress. These factors mainly include patient's symptoms, functional status and duration of illness (Cook, Lefley, Pickett & Cohler, 1994; Cuijpers, 1999), and caregiver's characteristics such as age, gender, hours of weekly contact with the patient, and kinship relations (Reinhard, 1994). Reported mediating factors include social support and coping skills (Solomon & Draine, 1995). In addition, family variables such as dysfunctional family roles and relationships, problematic communication patterns, family conflicts, and incongruence of family members' appraisal of the patient can also exacerbate caregiver burden (Lemmens et al., 2003). As suggested by Maurin and Boyd (1990), the beliefs held by family members regarding what factors influence events and situations during the course of schizophrenia are also important factors in determining how well family caregivers cope with caring for the patient.

One limitation of the concept of family burden is its connotation of negative emotions, whereas many caregivers find their role fulfilling and uplifting (Bland & Darlington, 2002). The dissonance between objective burden and subjective satisfaction with the caregiving experience has been noted in the literature (Martens & Addington, 2001), and has resulted in the suggestion that the "experience of caregiving" or "psychological well-being" of family caregivers should replace the use of "caregiver burden." However, the negative effects of caregiving on family functioning, daily routines, and physical and psychological well-being of family members of patients with severe mental illness are noteworthy, and, most importantly, so are the false beliefs about and social stigma towards mental illness in Chinese and other Asian countries (Ma & Yip, 1997; Meredith et al., 1994). Therefore, although there is no widely-accepted theoretical framework of family burden, it is important to understand that caring for a relative with schizophrenia and other severe mental illnesses imposes a feeling of burden on family caregivers (Rungreangkulkij & Gilliss, 2000).

*Chapter 4*

# IMPORTANCE OF FAMILY INTERVENTION FOR CLIENTS WITH SCHIZOPHRENIA

There are several reasons for providing interventions to families of people with schizophrenia. First, studies on expressed emotion—which refers to the critical or emotionally over-involved attitudes and behavior displayed by one or more family members regarding their relative with schizophrenia (Kavanagh, 1995)—have revealed that family dynamics and emotional climate affect the reoccurrence of positive symptoms and, therefore, the course of the illness (Butzlaff & Hooley, 1998). While the mechanisms of action of high expressed emotion in the course of schizophrenia are unclear, it is clear that a high level of distress is inevitably experienced by a patient who is in regular and frequent contact with such family members (Mueser & Gingerich, 1994; Repper & Brooker, 1998). However, the education and involvement of these family members in the planning and implementation of treatment can only benefit the monitoring of progress of treatment and changes in patient's condition. Enhanced ability of family members to detect any warning signs of relapse, and notifying health professionals about such signs, can be crucial in preventing these illness relapses. There have been reports of long delays in treatment due to inadequate family support (Barnes et al., 2000; Drake et al., 2000).

Second, having an intimate relationship with a relative with schizophrenia and providing care for such a person can induce a great burden on family members. Families, if used as a "dumping ground" for these patients, may be overwhelmed by the challenges and difficulties in managing a patient with schizophrenia (Iodice & Wodarski, 1987), even though there are some positive aspects of caregiving, such as a sense of inner strength and satisfaction, personal growth and enhanced family relationships (Greenberg, Greenley & Benedict,

1994; Mueser, 2003). Reducing caregiver burden is an important goal of family support and care that can help family members remain involved with their loved ones while maintaining their own psychological and physical well-being (Mueser, 2003).

Lastly, high levels of stress within a family, which may arise from caregiver burden, can have a negative effect on a patient's illness, increasing their vulnerability to relapse (Butzlaff & Hooley, 1998). The intimate relationship and interactions between patients with schizophrenia and their family members warrant application of family-centred interventions for improving the ability of families to work with their patient to cope more effectively with stress relating to caregiving from within and outside the family (Mueser & Glynn, 1999).

Families were once scapegoated as a major causative factor of the pathogenesis of schizophrenia (Lefley, 1996), but the weight of evidence today is that families can play a vital role in helping their relatives with schizophrenia make good progress towards their recovery (Mueser, 2003). Working with families would appear to be one effective way of delivering community-based intervention to the patients. Nevertheless, families need adequate support themselves if they are to support their disabled relative. To enhance family support and care for patients with schizophrenia, there has been an increase in the number of research studies on developing and testing different modes of family intervention over the past 20 years. Therefore, the following chapter draws on the literature on the development and major types of family intervention for patients with schizophrenia and their theoretical basis, and looks at the evidence supporting their relative effectiveness for these patients and their families.

*Chapter 5*

# DEVELOPMENT OF FAMILY INTERVENTIONS

Treatments for patients with schizophrenia reflect dominant ideas on the causes of the illness. The origins of family intervention can be traced to theories of family causation of the illness, which go back to the 1940s and 1950s. In the 1950s, research on dysfunctional communication in families originated from the idea of the "double bind" (Bateson et al., 1956), which occurs when an instruction is given overtly to a patient by family members, but is contradicted by a second more covert instruction. As suggested by Bateson, this double bind communication leaves the child able to make only ambiguous or meaningless responses, and schizophrenia was thought to develop when this process persists. Studies of communication in families of patients with schizophrenia have indicated rather inconsistent and conflicting findings (Hirsch & Leff, 1975). The disordered family communication and role relationships are considered to be important factors associated with the course of the illness and the patient's recovery.

In the late 1950s, the theory of expressed emotions (EE) was developed in an attempt to describe emotional attitudes of family members towards patients with schizophrenia and its relationship with the illness. The concept of EE was developed by Brown et al. (1962) and measured with a semi-structured interview schedule (Camberwell Family Interview) on three dimensions: criticisms, hostility, and emotional involvement. This EE concept has proven useful for understanding the interactions within families with a member suffering from schizophrenia. A meta-analysis by Butzlaff and Hooley (1998) of 27 studies of the EE-outcome relationship with schizophrenia in the U.S. and other Western countries confirmed that EE is a significant and robust predictor of relapse in schizophrenia (i.e., the weighted mean effect size was 0.31), particularly for those primary family caregivers with high face-to-face contact with the patient. More evidence continues to accumulate highlighting the link between the health status of patients and family caregivers and family relationships (Cole & Reiss, 1993; Wearden et al., 2000).

Leff and Vaughn (1985), using a combination of support and education for family members, managed to successfully lower expressed emotion in families and thus positively reduce patients' relapse rate (i.e., 14% relapse in family support group vs. 78% in control group with regular medications over two-year follow-up). Since then, EE-related research has focused not only on the patient's relapse but also on the effect of caregiving on the whole family. Karanci and Inandilar's (2002) study of coping and distress of caregivers of Turkish patients with schizophrenia indicated that caregivers' perceptions of their ability to cope with the patient's symptomatic behaviors, such as aggression and antisocial behavior, and their reported distress due to these behaviors, are closely related to their EE level. Similarly, in the U.K., Budd, Oles and Hughes (1998) studied the relationship between caregiver burden and coping style in 91 caregivers of patients with schizophrenia and reported that emotional over-involvement and criticism are associated with higher levels of family burden. It has also resulted in various therapeutic and educational strategies aimed at reducing family caregivers' EE in order to improve patients' illness and symptom intensity, and thus reduce relapse rates.

A long-standing theoretical rationale underlying the use of family-centered interventions comes from studies in the West, which have reported consistently that patients with schizophrenia who live in families that have high levels of EE have relapse rates three to 10 times greater than those who live in low EE families (Bebbington & Kuipers, 1994; Ivanovic, Vuletic & Bebbington, 1994). Studies on EE also showed that the role of family attitudes and interactions influenced the course of schizophrenia, but there was insufficient evidence that it influenced onset of the illness, as might be predicted by the stress-vulnerability model (Kavanagh, 1995; Barrowclough & Johnston, 1996; Wearden et al., 2000). Barrowclough and Parle (1997) suggest that critical factors common to successful psychosocial intervention for schizophrenia include helping the family, especially those with high levels of EE, to reduce their negative attitudes towards the patient's illness and increase their confidence in coping with the patient's symptoms and bizarre behavior.

Family intervention techniques have developed gradually and become accepted as an alternative to biomedical or pharmacological treatment for changing families' attitudes, relationships, and communication patterns. However, even up to the late 1970s, family theories and therapies for schizophrenia were supported by little empirical evidence. Most studies showed disappointing, non-significant or modest results, which contrasted with over-ambitious claims for the efficacy of family therapy. Anderson and Adams (1996) and Dixon et al. (1999) suggest that, in the West, there are difficulties in employing family intervention in everyday clinical practice with groups of patients with schizophrenia in receipt of community care due to inadequate mental health care services, staff training and resources. Research in the 1980s has already indicated that information and caregiving skills learning were important but were too frequently unavailable as a community resource for patients and families (Noh & Turner, 1987). A field study in the U.S. (Dixon et al., 1999) also found that less than one-third of patients who have contact with their families reported that their families had received information, support, or advice about their illness and less than 10% said that their families had attended an educational or supportive program. Ma and Yip (1997) suggest similar reasons to explain why family intervention has not been frequently used in community-based treatment for patients with schizophrenia in Hong Kong and other Chinese populations.

In spite of inadequately trained therapists, research over the 1980s has established a more sound evidence base on the effects of family environment for schizophrenia, especially for those families with highly critical or emotionally over-involved attitudes towards patients. Owing to greatly increased interest and understanding of the importance of the role of the family in caring for patients with schizophrenia in the community, there have been very positive advances in the development of different types of family intervention in parallel to psychosocial intervention for patients with schizophrenia over the last 15 years (Brooker, 2001; Mueser, 2003). Demands for family interventions within the community have also increased substantially as a result of changes in the organization of mental health services over the past decade in Western countries (Budd et al., 1998) as well as in Hong Kong. It is beyond a doubt that the current emphasis on community care and caring for the caregivers has made family intervention a crucial component of the treatment plans for patients with schizophrenia. Wide dissemination of an effective model of family intervention is a priority for improvement of contemporary community mental health services.

Pharoah et al. (2001) and Pilling et al. (2002), in their meta-analysis of controlled trials of family interventions involving more than 2,000 patients with schizophrenia (from 1980 to 1999) in different countries such as the U.S., the U.K., Australia, and mainland China, concluded that all types of family intervention (both single and group format) are more effective in reducing patient relapse up to one year, readmission up to two years, and rates of treatment compliance when compared to standard care. As recommended by the American Psychiatric Association (1997) and Schizophrenia Patient Outcomes Research Team (Lehman, Steinwachs & the Survey Co-investigators of the PORT Project, 1998), which was funded by the National Institute of Mental Health in the U.S., patients who have ongoing contact with their families should be offered a family psychosocial intervention that spans at least six months and provides a combination of education about the illness, family support, crisis intervention, and problem-solving skills training. In addition, the team suggests that family intervention should not be restricted to patients whose families are identified as having high levels of expressed emotion. Similarly, the National Institute for Clinical Excellence in the U.K., in its clinical guideline of core interventions in the management of patients with schizophrenia, suggests that family intervention should be available to the families who are living with or who are in close contact with patients with schizophrenia (National Collaborating Centre for Mental Health, 2002).

Nevertheless, the past decade has witnessed the rapid growth of a variety of family intervention strategies, which have been largely influenced by cognitive-behavioral and stress and crisis theories. Single or multiple-family group intervention programs and those consisting mainly of educational, behavioral, and supportive components have been used in the treatment of people with a variety of chronic mental health problems such as depression, anxiety disorders (Anderson, Reiss & Hogarty, 1986), dementia (McCallion & Toseland, 1995), and eating disorders (Dare & Eisler, 2000). However, different terms are used to refer to work with families, such as psycho-educational, psychosocial, family education, family management, family support, or combinations of these terms. In the absence of agreed terminology, the guidelines suggested by Fadden (1998) in the research update on family interventions may be helpful. Fadden suggested that the terms psychosocial, psycho-education, and behavioral management approaches to family interventions generally refer to those interventions in an individual or group format in which the patient and family members meet together; such a format includes a component of skills acquisition in addition to a didactic teaching element and the primary aim of the program is to reduce patient relapse and readmission. He also suggested that family education, consultation, support and counseling and relatives' groups usually refer to interventions directed at family members (excluding the patient), and their primary focus is on addressing the needs of family members. Nevertheless, these family education and consultation programs are not frequently used or fairly and consistently structured, and the families in the programs meet the therapist on an irregular schedule or whenever in need. They have proven to be much less effective and acceptable in current practice. Fadden's suggestions are helpful in providing a background for the description of the major types of family intervention and their relative effectiveness for families of patients with schizophrenia, which are to be described in the following chapter.

*Chapter 6*

# TYPES OF FAMILY INTERVENTION AND THEIR EFFECTIVENESS

Four board modes of family intervention are frequently used in the West and mainland China to address specific treatment outcomes including reduction of patient relapse and family burden and improvement of family and patient functioning. These modes include family psycho-education, behavioral family management, multiple-family group intervention, and family consultation or supportive counseling. The empirical bases of these four modes of intervention are defined, described and discussed. They are also compared in terms of their relative effectiveness based on the previous literature.

## FAMILY PSYCHO-EDUCATIONAL PROGRAMS

The psycho-educational model of family care conceptualized by the pioneers focuses on the plight of people with mental illness, particularly on the higher risk of relapse and re-hospitalization, which come at great a cost to the patient and to society as a whole (Anderson et al., 1986; Falloon, Body & McGill, 1984). These researchers posited that family behavior plays an important role in patient functioning and that families can be educated to create an environment in which relapse can be reduced. Family psycho-education is the most frequently-used model of family intervention for patients with schizophrenia in Western countries as well as in Asian countries (Dixon, Adams & Luckstead, 2000). In the 1980s, these programs of family intervention were initiated in response to the effect of expressed emotion in families of patients with schizophrenia on patient relapse, assisting these family members to enhance their ability to cope with the illness (Dixon et al., 2000). Over the past 20 years, several modes of family psycho-education for schizophrenia have been developed and empirically tested. The theoretical foundations for these interventions are mainly derived from stress and coping models and other psychological theories such as cognitive-behavioral, social learning and crisis theories (Lukens, Thorning & Herman, 1999). According to Lukens et al. (1999). Psycho-educational intervention grows naturally out of the framework of stress reduction and adaptation because it implies that coping with difficult family caregiving situations requires family members to have knowledge, coping skills, and adequate psychosocial support. Since psycho-education interventions focus mainly on the patient's mental condition, studies in family psycho-education have given limited attention to family burden and to family perceptions of problems and needs (Hatfield, 1994).

While family psycho-education broadly characterizes a range of approaches to educational intervention for families of patients with schizophrenia, there are several features common to the effective programs, including structural components, philosophical perspectives, goals, and content. First, their common structural components are the following: the programs are designed and led by health professionals; they are long-term, lasting between nine months to two years; they are an integral part of the patient's treatment plan along with medication and other psychiatric treatments; they may be delivered to single or multiple families at the patient's home or in a clinical setting; and they include both the family members and the patient during the intervention sessions (Dixon et al., 2000). Second, the philosophical perspectives of these interventions emphsize the here-and-now circumstances and improving the future, while avoiding delving into the past and imposing blame (Mueser, 2003). The treatment team seeks to establish a collaborative relationship with the family in order to share the burden of managing the illness and working towards patient recovery. Lastly, in terms of goals and content, all programs focus on providing information about the illness and its treatment, management the patient's illness behavior, problem-solving and coping skills in caregiving, and access to family support services (Lehman et al., 1998). Such information is crucial for family caregivers to cope with the caregiving role.

## Behavioral Family Management

Behavioral family management (BFM) for patients with schizophrenia was developed by Falloon, Liberman, Lillie and Vaughan (1981) in the U.S. using family education, training in communication skills and practice in problem solving. This program, delivered in the context of multiple-family groups and held for 10 sessions over a three-month period, was shown to have beneficial effects for the patients (Falloon & Liberman, 1983). This intervention has been refined, elaborated and implemented across a wide variety of socio-economic and cultural groups in the U.S., U.K., and mainland China (Falloon et al., 1985; McFarlane et al., 1995; Montero et al., 2001; Xiong et al., 1994), proving effective in reducing symptoms, promoting remission, strengthening social functioning, and reducing family burden. This intervention is based on a functional analysis of the family and the application of learning principles and problem-solving techniques to help family members learn how to manage patients with schizophrenia in collaboration with mental health professionals (Falloon, Boyd & McGill, 1984). Because the behavioral approach assumes that the patient, family, therapist, and other elements of the mental health services are interactive and open to change at different levels, families of patients with schizophrenia should be assisted to understand their own specific needs at different points in time to achieve the ultimate goal of comprehensive and continuous care of the patients (Hatfield, 1994). Behavioral family therapists conduct ongoing thorough assessments of the needs, assets, deficits, burden, stress, and desires of these family members and assist them in setting goals of learning to better cope with caregiving, solving problems, and communicating more directly and constructively with the patient and other family members.

BFM has been operationalized to the point at which its procedures are now available in a detailed and clearly-described treatment manual and a workbook, which serve as the foundation for the family's effective management of the illness. Different modes of the BFM program range from 10 to 20 sessions and span from six months to two years (Mueser & Gylnn, 1999).

According to Mueser and Gylnn (1999), the BFM programs mainly consist of six components: engaging (introduction of the program and exploration of the benefits of family work, followed by initial discussion about family problems); assessment (individual interviews with family members to gather information about the illness, family background, and their personal goals in participation in the program from the perspective of each family member and to establish a trusting relationship with the therapist); psycho-education (information about the illness, treatment, medication compliance, the role of the family in caregiving, and improvement in the patient's independence and recovery); communication skills training (improvement of the ability of family members to communicate in direct, effective, and non-stressful ways); problem-solving training (teaching family members a standardized approach for helping them face problems in caregiving and collaboratively identifying alternative solutions to the problems); and the termination phase (a discussion of the family's accomplishments, community resources, and future plans).

## MULTIPLE-FAMILY GROUP INTERVENTIONS

Multiple-family education groups are a professional-led intervention in a group format aimed at providing continued education and support for people with schizophrenia and other severe mental illnesses and their family members, and are usually provided on a time-unlimited basis (Mueser & Glynn, 1999). These groups are more economical than single-family educational intervention and consultation, providing more opportunities for social support among participants, and providing a forum for continued psycho-education about the nature and management of schizophrenia (Mueser, 2003). However, there are different types of multiple-family groups, such as family-dynamic multi-family groups in New Jersey (Marsh, 1998; McFarlane et al., 1995), and family-aided assertive community treatment in New York (McFarlane, Stastny & Deakins, 1992; Stein & Santos, 1998). Most of them are based on the family psycho-education or behavioral model, but each intervention has its emphasis on the techniques and objectives of intervention. For example, the family-dynamic multi-family groups (Marsh, 1998) emphasized opening intra-family communication, sharing emotional responses and attempting to resolve family conflicts. The therapists did not provide any education about schizophrenia and medication compliance, and did not use any structured problem-solving techniques. The family-aided assertive community treatment integrated systematic and ongoing family psycho-education or family crisis intervention and an intensive case management approach (McFarlane et al., 1992), specifically targeting the less treatment-responsive group of patients with schizophrenia. Supportive family management developed by Zastowny, Lehman, Cole and Kane (1992) in New York for a highly treatment-resistant population of young adults with chronic schizophrenia provides patients and families with detailed information about the illness and treatment plan, and direct advice to families concerning linkage to community resources and management of crises and day-to-day patient and family difficulties. Brief family therapy techniques are also employed to support the families when indicated and serve to help them treasure their caregiving role.

As suggested by McFarlane (2002) and Mueser (2003), multiple-family groups are guided by five important goals: (1) educating family members about mental illness and its treatment; (2) establishing and promoting social support for patients and families; (3) training in problem-solving skills to address common difficulties and distress; (4) sharing and practicing patient management strategies; and (5) providing information on and access to community resources and consultation for family support.

## FAMILY EDUCATION, CONSULTATION OR SUPPORTIVE COUNSELING

Family consultation, sometimes called supportive family counseling, is an individualized approach of support and education to a family member or the whole family of a patient with schizophrenia (Bernheim, 1987; Marsh & Johnson, 1997). It focuses on the adaptive strengths of a family rather than its pathology and deficits. The consultant may be either a health professional with expertise in family counseling or a trained family member who provides information and advice to family members as needed on the mental illness, mental status assessment, mediation strategies, problem management, and referrals to community resources (Marsh & Johnson, 1997). The intervention is a flexible approach, which is collaboration between the family and consultant to determine the goals and plan of action; it is a very short-term educational intervention for families whose ill relatives refuse or resist treatment (Bernheim, 1987).

Similar to other family consultation programs, Solomon et al.'s (1996) study reported on an individual family consultation conducted by the Training and Education Centre Network in the U.S., a collaborative initiative of mental health professionals and family members experienced in providing family education to individuals with a mentally ill relative. The program provided a minimum of six hours of consultation to each family, including a two-hour assessment, at least two hours of face-to-face contact, and at least two additional hours of either face-to-face or telephone contact. The maximum amount of service was 15 hours. Families determined the focus of their education with their consultant and could contact the consultant on an as-needed basis. Generally, family consultation was a time-limited intervention, from two to three months and from 15 to 30 hours of contact with the family, and thus was only focused on one or two specific objectives. As suggested by Solomon (1996), this intervention was effective in improving families' knowledge of or insight into the illness and medications as well as patients' medication compliance.

Family education programs, either in individual or group format, are usually short in duration (from one day to less than six months) and focus on providing families of people with schizophrenia with information on mental illness and advice on its management (Biegel, Robinson & Kennedy, 2000). This type of intervention may be led by mental health professionals or by trained peer leaders. Family education also adopts a strengths perspective, in which families are encouraged and assisted to develop their stress management and coping skills and to improve their psychological well-being and ability to adapt to dealing with their relative's illness (Solomon, 2000). Many of the family education programs have been developed by families in response to their dissatisfaction with the information and support that health professionals have offered to them; these families often feel that they need practical, hands-on assistance with day-to-day problems instead of only standardized medical treatment and care (Hatfield, 1994).

*Chapter 7*

# Commonalities of Different Modes of Family Intervention

Most recently-developed family intervention programs begin with a few teaching sessions, which cover basic information on the etiology, symptoms, medical and psychological treatments, and prognosis of schizophrenia (McFarlane, 2002; Pilling et al., 2002; Hazel et al., 2004). Intervention approaches differ in subsequent sessions over content, format, duration, and the time intervals between sessions. As suggested by the Schizophrenia Patients Outcomes Research Team in the U.S. (Lehman et al., 1998), family education and support programs are usually organized around the central theme of providing family members of people with schizophrenia with education about the illness and its treatment, guidance and resources for patient care and for family caregivers during crisis, and training in managing common problems in caregiving. Even though different techniques or approaches are used, family interventions for schizophrenia aims to achieve some common goals, including (1) working in alliance with families who care for the person with schizophrenia to identify stressors associated with family dysfunction and patient relapse; (2) enhancement of problem anticipation and problem solving; (3) improvement of family atmosphere by reduction of high emotional involvement and critical attitudes towards the patient by their family, such as hostility and criticism; (4) setting realistic expectations on the patient's social and vocational concerns and performance in the home; (5) helping families improve communication and relationship with patients; and (6) attainment of desirable change in family members' behavior and understanding of the illness and its care (Pharoah et al., 2001; Thornicroft & Susser, 2001). However, little is known about the therapeutic value of different components or strategies (Dyck et al., 2002). With better understanding of these crucial therapeutic elements within family intervention, it may be possible to develop a more consistent, reliable, and effective family intervention program for patients with schizophrenia.

In addition, two reviews of family intervention studies (Dixon et al., 2000; Solomon, 2000) suggest that there are several characteristics common to the four modes of family intervention mentioned above: leadership and delivery by health professionals such as nurses, social workers, and psychiatrists; primary focus on patient outcomes such as relapse and medication compliance with family outcomes as secondary; primary focus on information about the illness, its medication and treatment, and strategies for patient management; involvement all interested family members, including the patient; more effective long-term intervention (e.g. at least six months); and exclusion of any beliefs and concepts that presume families are the causal agent of the development of schizophrenia.

## Relative Effectiveness of Different Modes of Family Intervention

A number of reviews from the mid 1990s, such as Barbato and D'Avanzo (2000), Mari and Streiner (1996) and Pilling et al. (2002), conducted in several countries—such as the U.S., the U.K. and other European countries, and mainland China—highlighted the possible advantages of family interventions for people with schizophrenia. Among the different models of family intervention in schizophrenia, psycho-education (e.g., Hogarty et al., 1991) and behavioral family management programs (e.g., Falloon et al., 1981) have been the most extensively studied modalities. More recently, needs-based psychosocial interventions (e.g., Sellwood et al., 2001) have been established with specific consideration of individual family needs.

However, there were some exceptions, namely, trials mostly undertaken in the 1970s and 1980s using models such as the crisis intervention model by Goldstein et al. (1978) and the psychodynamic model by Kottgen et al. (1984). These models demonstrated negative or non-significant effects when compared with standard care (Leff & Vaughn, 1985; Levene et al., 1989) or psycho-education intervention (McFarlane et al., 1995), and evaluations suffered major methodological limitations such as small sample size, non-equivalent or no control group, and case study design.

A relatively recent systematic review of controlled trials between 1978 and 1996 by the Cochrane Schizophrenia Group (Pharoah et al., 2001) suggests that most psycho-education and supportive approaches of family intervention have consistently demonstrated positive effects on reducing patients' relapse rate and improving patients' medication compliance and families' knowledge about the illness. The specific effects of family intervention on family members' psychosocial needs, such as family functioning, coping with caregiving, psychological distress and burden of care, and management of the patient within the home environment, have not been studied adequately, and so data are few and equivocal. However, those few studies (Falloon et al., 1981; Tarrier, 1991; Xiong et al., 1994) that have included an economic evaluation suggest that psycho-educational or behavioral family intervention is more cost-effective than conventional mental health care services.

When comparing the effects of different models of family intervention on patient and family outcomes, studies in mainland China (Xiong et al., 1994; Zhang et al., 1994), the U.K. (Tarrier et al., 1994), and other Western countries (Dixon et al., 2001; McFarlane, Dixon, Lukens & Lucksted, 2003) have consistently demonstrated that family psycho-education and/or behavioral approaches of intervention spanning at least 10 sessions over six months are more effective and show relatively long-lasting effects (more than three years) on the prevention of relapse among people with schizophrenia than individual psychosocial treatment or medication alone. However, the psycho-education and behavioral approaches of intervention, as described by researchers in previous studies, consisted of a variety of content, format, and techniques. The common elements in several approaches of effective family psycho-education programs include social support, education about the illness and its treatment, guidance and resources during crisis, and training in problem solving (Dixon et al., 2000; Lehman & Steinwachs, 1998). However, little is known about the major therapeutic components of psycho-education and other psychosocial family interventions for schizophrenia (Barbato & D'Avanzo, 2000).

## EVIDENCE ON THE EFFECTIVENESS OF FAMILY PSYCHO-EDUCATION

Over the past 20 years, the psycho-education approaches to family intervention have been used most frequently and evaluated in trials to be most efficacious in Western and Asian countries, and the findings of these studies add to our knowledge of family intervention. Some specific points are important for research and practice. First, when compared with other models of family intervention, psycho-education intervention is most effective in reducing patient relapse and readmission; this finding is robust across cultures (e.g., Leff (1994) in the U.K.; Xiong et al. (1994) in mainland China; McFarlane et al. (1995) in the U.S.; Canive et al. (1996) in Spain; Chou, Liu & Chu (2002) in Taiwan), sustainable over time up to eight years (Tarrier et al., 1994), and can reduce costs of care (Xiong et al., 1994).

Second, offering psycho-education to multiple families in groups, and including the patients, has been found to be highly effective, especially when some patients have florid positive psychotic symptoms (McFarlane, 2002; Pilling et al., 2002). However, there are two important issues that the service providers should consider. (1) Multiple-family groups may have very high non-compliance or attrition rates due to group members' time constraints imposed by work and domestic life, and inconvenience of transport and meeting times and the impact of these factors on attending groups; moreover, they may not be able to temporarily settle the patient in a safe place and arrange for alternative care for the patient when attending the group (Chien, Chan, Morrissey & Thompson, 2005; Vaughan et al., 1992). (2) Running a family group requires a highly-skilled and experienced therapist who can effectively manage numbers of patients with active psychotic symptoms and disturbing behavior, along with their highly-distressed family caregivers (Fadden, 1998).

Third, the focus of intervention is usually on family education and problem-solving skills training to develop families' coping skills in tackling day-to-day problems. Studies comparing family psycho-education with psychodynamic or counseling approaches indicate that psycho-education intervention is more effective in improving families' knowledge and coping skills for caregiving (Vaughan et al., 1992; McFarlane, 1994). However, providing information or education alone without a skills training component only benefits family caregivers' satisfaction with mental health services and increases their knowledge about the illness and its treatment (Posner et al., 1992), but has been shown to have only a short-term or insignificant effect on patient relapse (Dixon et al., 2000). Family education is likely to be an important component for engagement of families in the intervention, and is best provided in the early stage of the illness when families can be assisted to develop correct concepts of the illness and positive beliefs regarding caregiving (Sidley, Smith & Howells, 1991).

Finally, brief crisis-oriented family psycho-education (Leff, 1994; Linszen et al., 1996) focusing on stress management and problem solving is more likely to be effective in relation to families' coping ability and patients' symptom control for families with low expressed emotion and those of patients experiencing their first psychotic episode when compared with detailed, lengthy psycho-education or behavioral intervention.

## EVIDENCE ON THE EFFECTIVENESS OF BEHAVIORAL MANAGEMENT PROGRAMS

Following Falloon et al.'s (1982) work on manual-driven behavioral family therapy for people with schizophrenia under community case management in the U.S., which showed a positive substantial effect on patient relapse and symptom control, there is now considerable evidence that different modes of problem-focused behavioral family interventions for patients with schizophrenia result in reduced relapse over one to two years' follow-up (Pharoah et al., 2001; Sellwood et al., 2001). Tarrier et al. (1989) conducted a controlled trial in the U.K. comparing the effect of a nine-month behavioral family intervention with a short educational program or routine treatment, which indicated that patient relapse within the behavioral intervention group was significantly lower than that of the other two groups at two-year follow-up. The findings of Berglund, Vahlne and Edman's (2003) study in Sweden also supported the assertion that behavioral family intervention reduced patient relapse and family burden and negative attitude towards caregiving when compared with conventional family support. A more recent trial of a needs-based and behavioral family intervention using Barrowclough and Tarrier's (1992) approach in the U.K. (Sellwood et al., 2001), indicated that family intervention based on a formal assessment of the family caregiver's needs was more effective in reducing patient relapse and caregiver's needs and improving patient functioning and positive symptoms over one-year follow-up when compared with routine family support and patient care. However, the researchers concluded that there were limited significant benefits for family caregivers participating in the behavioral intervention, as well as no improvement in patients' medication compliance.

Telles et al. (1995) compared the effectiveness and cross-cultural applicability of Falloon's behavioral management program and standard case management in symptom reduction, functional status and illness relapse of 40 low-income Spanish-speaking people with schizophrenia in the U.S. over one year. The results of this evaluation did not support the positive findings of previous studies when applied to a socio-cultural diverse population. Hence, socio-cultural factors may influence family members' responses to different types of family intervention. These findings also raise the question of whether a behavioral family management program can be applied effectively to socio-culturally diverse populations.

The Treatment Strategies for Schizophrenia study (Schooler et al., 1997), in a sample of more than 200 patients with schizophrenia in the U.S., reported that there was no significant difference in patients' medication compliance and readmission over 24-month follow-up between behavioral family intervention and supportive multiple-family group intervention, although both approaches appeared to have a positive effect on these outcomes. Bellack, Haas, Schooler and Flory (2000) continued the Treatment Strategies for Schizophrenia study and reported that the intensive behavioral intervention did not result in a more significant improvement in family communication and problem-solving ability than supportive family intervention over the two-year study period.

Similarly, Zastowny, Lehman, Cole and Kane (1992) in New York also reported that behavioral family treatment following Falloon's approach did not show significantly greater improvements in patients' functional status, symptom control and re-hospitalization, or families' burden, functioning and problem-solving than that of supportive family management developed by Bernheim and Lehman (1985). Consistent with the findings of these studies, several recent reviews have raised questions about the importance of behavioral skills training and the mechanisms of therapeutic actions of family interventions and other psychosocial interventions (Dixon et al., 2000; Pharoah et al., 2001). Given the higher cost of intensive training and procedures of a behavioral family management program, Bellack et al. (2000), in their study of the effects of behavioral family management on family communication and patients' relapse and symptom management, suggested that less intensive, educational or supportive family interventions that can demonstrate similar positive effects for patients and families should be used in order to ensure choosing the more cost-effective family intervention for the patients. Although these studies do not support behavioral family management as being more effective than supportive and educational approaches of family intervention, it should be noted that these studies did not include a control group (standard care) for comparison of their relative effectiveness.

Overall, past studies in Western countries indicate that behavioral family intervention can produce significant positive effects on patient outcomes such as relapse and symptom control, but there were no significant positive effects on family caregivers' psychosocial conditions and problem solving. As suggested by reviews of trials in family interventions for people with schizophrenia (Barbato & D'Avanzo, 2000; Bustillo et al., 2001), behavioral family intervention, which consists of a clearly-defined set of behavioral techniques following a step-by-step skill-building format conducted by an intensively-trained professional, may not produce better patient and family-related outcomes when compared with other family educational and supportive interventions. There is no published study on behavioral family intervention within Chinese or Asian populations.

## EVIDENCE ON THE EFFECTIVENESS OF MULTIPLE-FAMILY GROUP INTERVENTIONS

In the 1980s, multiple-family group (MFG) interventions for people with schizophrenia were implemented in combination with different educational and behavioral approaches, but there were limited empirical trials of their effectiveness on patient and family-related outcomes. The recent commonly-used format of multiple-family group for people with schizophrenia—an ongoing, closed, long-term group led by at least two clinicians, involving both patients and their families—was evaluated in a few clinical trials by McFarlane and his colleagues in the U.S. in the 1990s. These studies demonstrated that multiple-family group interventions using psycho-education and/or behavioral approaches for first-episode and high-risk patients with schizophrenia or patients with highly stressed families are consistently more effective in improving patients' relapse and employment rate than single-family interventions. These positive patient outcomes of multi-family intervention increase with time, up to four years. McFarlane, Link, Dushay et al. (1995) conducted a three-group comparison among psycho-educational MFG, psycho-education in a single-family format, and MFG (mainly discussion and sharing facilitated by two clinicians during group meetings) without psycho-education for 41 inpatients with schizophrenia, using symptomatic relapse as the main outcome criterion. The respective relapse rates at four years were 50%, 78% and 57%, and the two MFGs reported similar relapse rate per year (12.5% for psycho-educational MFG and 14% for MFG without psycho-education). These results indicate that, when combined with antipsychotic medication, the MFGs with two different formats can produce a longer-term and more positive effect on patient relapse when compared with the single-family psycho-education group. Another clinical trial conducted by McFarlane, Stastny and Deakins (1992) examined the relative effect of psycho-educational MFG combined with assertive community treatment (termed family-aided assertive community treatment, FACT) and single-family crisis intervention (SCI) on 68 patients with schizophrenia with respect to their employment, re-hospitalization, symptoms (positive and negative), medication compliance, and family burden and well-being over a two-year follow-up. The psycho-educational MFG resulted in a significantly higher employment rate over two years (32% versus 19% for SCI). While there were no significance differences between the two groups for the other four outcomes, the two groups demonstrated similar significant improvements in these four aspects over the two years (about 38% of the baseline symptom severity, a reduction of chlorpromazine equivalents from 975 mg to 696 mg, an increase in median medication compliance from 75% to 100%, and improvements in families' ratings of objective and subjective burden).

The New York Family Psycho-Education Study compared an MFG and a single-family intervention over two years at five state psychiatric hospitals and one city hospital using a large representative sample of patients with schizophrenia (Marsh, 1994), and reported that the patients' relapse rate for the MFG was exactly one-third less than that of the single-family intervention (27.7% versus 41.6%). In addition, the Caucasian patients in the MFG who did not fully remit on medication and had a family member with high expressed emotion displayed a significantly lower relapse rate than those in the single-family intervention group (9% versus 56%) and the African-American patients in the two interventions (42% for MFG and 22% for single-family intervention). Mean dosage of antipsychotic medication in the MFG decreased over two years, whereas the mean dosage increased in the single-family intervention. The consistent positive effect of MFG on patients' relapse reported in these studies regardless of the content and approach of intervention used may be explained by the expansion of families' social network and increase of peer support resulting from group participation. Further research is needed to examine the importance of social support and other therapeutic components in the MFG intervention.

Hazel et al. (2004) in the U.S. compared the effects of an MFG treatment (n = 53) using McFarlane's approach and standard care (n = 44) for people with schizophrenia or schizoaffective disorder and demonstrated that the MFG significantly reduced family caregivers' distress when compared with standard care over two years. However, there were no significant differences in families' psychosocial support resources between the two groups after two years. This may be due to the limited amount of time per month the participants devoted to multiple-family group treatment, which was not sufficient to allow for a significant increase in social support. Moreover, as pointed out by McDonell et al. (2003), multiple-family psycho-education groups for patients with schizophrenia might not reduce family burden because the group intervention focused on patients' illness management and recovery, but not on family caregivers' psychological well-being and support resources.

As a result, there is relatively less research reporting that MFG intervention for people with schizophrenia indicates greater positive effects on family-related outcomes such as burden and other psychosocial functioning than other modes of single- and multiple-family interventions. Among a few studies supporting the benefits of MFG to family caregivers, Dyck et al. (2000) in Spokane, Washington demonstrated a more postive effect of a psycho-educational MFG using McFarlane's approach for 63 outpatients with schizophrenia at a large community mental health centre on caregivers' physical health compared with standard care. A lower percentage of caregivers in MFG (23%) visited their physicians more than once compared with the standard care group (31%) over the 12-month follow-up period. Results of stepwise regression analysis also indicated that treatment group, together with onset of illness and number of pre-intervention physician visits, predicted the number of post-intervention physician visits ($p < 0.05$).

However, other clinical trials in Western countries indicate that there is no significant difference between multiple-family group intervention and single-family mode of intervention for people with schizophrenia in both patient and family-related outcomes such as relapse rates and patient and family functioning. Leff et al. (1990) in London, U.K. also conducted a trial to compare the effect between individual family therapy (12 families that included patients), a supportive family education group (11 families that excluded patients), and routine care for patients with schizophrenia in families with high expressed emotion. Patients' relapse rates in the individual family therapy and supportive family group (33% and 36%) were similar and significantly lower than the relapse rate for the families under routine care (about 75%) at two-year follow-up. In Hogarty et al.'s (1997) psycho-educational MFG study using Anderson, Reiss and Hogarty's (1986) approach (versus single-family personal therapy, single-family supportive therapy, and a combination of MFG and personal therapy) for 97 patients with schizophrenia or schizoaffective disorder in the U.S., those patients receiving personal therapy alone showed a significantly lower psychotic relapse rate (28%) than either the supportive therapy or family therapy patient (38% and 45%) over three-year follow-up. However, 13 of 15 treatment-related terminations among the patients living with family occurred in the no-personal-therapy category, particularly under the condition of supportive therapy, thus limiting survivorship to less representative and possibly less vulnerable patients in these no-personal-therapy conditions.

In addition, some clinical trials in the U.S. and U.K. demonstrate that there are no significant differences between different approaches of multiple-family group intervention for people with schizophrenia in patient and family-related outcomes. In the U.S., Zastowny et al. (1992) and Schooler et al. (1997) compared the effects of two approaches of multiple-family group intervention—Falloon's approach of behavioral family management and supportive counseling with educational workshops—on patients' relapse, re-hospitalization and dosage of antipsychotic medication over two years. The findings of these two studies indicated that there were no significant differences in patients' relapse and dosage of medication between the two approaches of multiple-family intervention. In the

U.K., Leff et al. (1989) also demonstrated that there were no significant improvements in symptomatic relapse and level of expressed emotion in both the family psycho-education group using the psychodynamic model and the supportive group intervention over two years.

Therefore, studies conducted in the U.K. and the U.S. over the past two decades demonstrate that multiple-family group interventions for people with schizophrenia using psycho-educational, behavioral, or other approaches indicate consistent positive effects on patients' relapse for up to four years. Most of these group programs included patients in the group meetings and consisted of an educational component and behavioral and problem-solving skills training. However, some limitations in studies on MFG have been pointed out as issues to address in future research. First, most research examined the effects of MFG on the patients' health condition, but less than half of the studies on MFG assessed families' health outcomes such as family burden, stress, and psychosocial functioning. Those few studies of MFG that have assessed the family-related outcomes have shown inconsistent findings or have failed to find marked improvements in family functioning or psychological well-being. Second, education and medication are necessary but not sufficient alone for improving patients' physical and psychosocial health conditions; other potential therapeutic components of group intervention should be explored for achieving better patient and/or family-related psychosocial outcomes.

As suggested by McFarlane (2002), the findings of clinical trials of MFGs in the U.S. in the 1990s support the conclusion that expansion of social network occurring in a long-term multiple-family group (meeting for at least six months) results in an increase of available social support, which may be a potentially important influence on treatment outcome. The importance of social support for families of people with chronic physical and mental illnesses has been well studied and has proven to be essential in contributing to psychological stability and a sense of social acceptance, and is thus associated with successful community tenure of patients with schizophrenia and other mental illnesses (Becker et al., 1998).

*Chapter 8*

# FAMILY INTERVENTION FOR PEOPLE WITH SCHIZOPHRENIA AND ITS LIMITATIONS

Despite inconsistent findings from studies of family intervention for schizophrenia, the superiority of family intervention over routine outpatient care has been demonstrated, and some significant effects such as relapse rate and medication compliance have been maintained for as long as two years. Recent reviews of more than 20 clinical trials of family intervention for people with schizophrenia conducted in Western countries and mainland China (Barbato & D'Avanzo, 2000; Dixon et al., 2000; Solomon, 2000; Pharoah et al., 2001) highlight questions about the effectiveness of family interventions which remain unanswered and require further research. First, there is a lack of conclusive evidence about the effects of commonly-used models of family intervention on health outcomes of family caregivers of people with schizophrenia. With much responsibility and burden placed on family members caring for their relative with schizophrenia under the trend of community care, more preparation of family caregivers in terms of knowledge and skills of caregiving, as well as coping with the illness and problems in caregiving, should be provided within the family intervention program. The family caregivers' psychosocial health conditions, which are significantly associated with the care of their ill relatives and the treatment outcomes, should be emphasized and treated as important indicators for the effectiveness of a family-focused intervention. Systematic assessment of family-related outcomes of family intervention including family functioning and burden, perceived social support, and health services utilization should also be demonstrated in future studies. In addition, Pharoah et al. (2001) suggested that there were clinically significant changes in family outcome measures following the intervention, which were defined and examined in this thesis to understand the significant and meaningful changes in psychosocial health conditions of family caregivers in the direction of functionality resulting from participation in the specifically designed family group work.

Second, little is known about the therapeutic value of different family intervention components or strategies. The described curative factors and mechanisms of change in the literature consist mainly of subjective accounts by therapists or facilitators of what they believed to be the important factors experienced within their own practice. Major identified factors include learning by analogy and identification of similar experience (Steinglass, 1998; Bishop et al., 2002), establishing a community of shared experiences (Steinglass, 1998), overcoming social stigma to the illness (Asen, 2002), and creating hope and adaptive patterns of coping and perspectives on illness and family life (Bishop et al., 2002). Although education about the illness and provision of social support are consistent ingredients of most models of family intervention for schizophrenia, they do not show any significant effect in isolation. Therefore, it is important to test the effect of family education and social support components in a specific model of family intervention emphasizing their use—for example, mutual support groups. In fact, mutual support groups have been used increasingly with patients with chronic physical diseases, terminal illnesses and enduring mental illness, and there is convincing evidence that they can meet caregivers' psychosocial needs (Cook et al., 1999). Further research is also needed to explore the most beneficial and important components of the family intervention used. The exploration of caregivers' perceived benefits and important therapeutic components of the intervention also comprise the major purpose of an evaluation study of a family mutual support group. With better understanding of these crucial therapeutic elements within the family intervention, it may be possible to develop a more consistent, reliable and effective family intervention program for patients with schizophrenia.

Third, previous studies examined the effects of the highly-structured family psycho-education model such as Anderson et al.'s (1986) family psycho-education program, and the manual-driven behavioral model such as Falloon et al.'s (1985) family behavioral management program. These studies indicated that these prevalent approaches of family intervention for people with schizophrenia did not show consistent immediate or long-term improvements in family members' psychosocial health conditions when compared with routine care or other simple supportive interventions, such as brief crisis-oriented family psycho-education (Leff, 1994; Linszen et al., 1996) and supportive family education programs (Bellack et al., 2000). Sellwood et al. (2001) also highlighted that effective family intervention may not require a specific defined set of advanced techniques delivered through a highly-structured model and manual of intervention, or with an intensively-trained professional. The positive results of their trial of a needs-based family intervention indicate that family intervention should be designed from a family caregiver's perspective to better recognize and meet their own psychosocial health needs in relation to caregiving, thus showing more positive family-related outcomes. In light of increasing empirical evidence in favor of multiple-family group interventions, bringing families together in supportive group intervention can produce specific and beneficial effects to family caregivers on improving their social support and coping with their caregiving role. The burden of care in schizophrenia is an issue that requires recognition, and attempts to ameliorate it rather than to provide support may be misplaced (Pilling et al., 2002).

Fourth, the implementation of family intervention techniques in routine practice has been hindered, however, for several reasons: most importantly, inadequate staff training and supervision, scarce resources, lack of availability of trained staff, and difficulty in maintaining the effectiveness of an intervention delivered over many years compared to a relatively short-term intervention which is subject to evaluation. Fadden (1998) shows great concern regarding implementation of family interventions in routine clinical practice, and suggests that many of the difficulties experienced most frequently by trained staff are related to service issues. For cognitive-behavioral family intervention to be effective, staff who are acting as therapists must be intensively trained and supervised in practice. It is often reported that trained staff cannot use the skills learned in their practice or intervention program following training without adequate supervision or management support (Kavanagh et al., 1993; Brooker, 2001). Also, therapists need to be able to work flexible hours in order to accommodate evening or weekend appointments. Those therapists who were able to visit families frequently reported that they only managed to do so by working on their own time or working outside regular hours. Dyck et al. (2002) suggested that running family intervention programs with multiple-family groups may be one way of overcoming these staff and resource limitations for individual family treatment.

Fifth, most of the studies of family intervention for people with schizophrenia were conducted in Western countries. The results of the evaluation of cross-cultural applicability of Falloon's behavioral management program in a Spanish-speaking population by Telles et al. (1995) did not support the positive findings from previous studies on patients' relapse and symptom control when applied to a socio-cultural diverse population. This finding indicates that socio-cultural factors may influence caregivers' responses to different types of family intervention.

Hence, modes of family intervention, which were originated in the West, should be tested in a variety of patient populations with different cultural backgrounds, thus providing more evidence of their relative effectiveness across cultures.

Finally, Barbato and D'Avanzo (2000), in their review of 25 clinical trials on family intervention, found that relapsed patients usually leave the trial and that trials too frequently fail to collect data on the period following relapses. This dropout or incomplete data collection is of particular concern for a long-term follow-up study. When designing a research study on family intervention, strategies such as asking for preferences and allowing more flexibility in time or convenience to attend the intervention sessions, and providing regular contact with and encouragement from the group and peer leaders between group meetings, should be built into the intervention in order to lower the attrition rate of the study.

*Chapter 9*

# EMERGENCE OF THE MUTUAL SUPPORT GROUP AS AN INTERVENTION FOR FAMILY CAREGIVERS

The proliferation of family mutual support groups in the United States and other Western countries in the 1980s is part of the larger social movement of self-help and mutual aid organizations for people affected by a variety of chronic diseases and stressful life circumstances, whose needs have been inadequately addressed by traditional health care interventions (Hatfield & Lefley, 1987; Heller, Roccoforte & Cook, 1997). Increasing research evidence has indicated that participation in a mutual support group for patients with different chronic physical and psychological problems—such as diabetes mellitus, bereavement and traumatic experiences, cancer and other terminal illnesses, and chronic mental illnesses—was highly associated with improvements in psychological adjustments of these patients (Spiegel et al., 1989; Zola, 1991) as well as family members (McCallion & Toseland, 1995). This growth in mutual support groups for patients led to an increasing interest in extending their use and examination of their value for family care of people with chronic physical and mental illnesses during the 1990s (Cook & Wright, 1996).

One influential and widely-held definition given by Katz et al. (1992) highlights eight important attributes that define a mutual support group. These are (a) an acknowledged purpose in coming together, more than mere social interaction; (b) voluntary participation with eagerness to regain normal life; (c) face-to-face small-group structure, usually between three to 12; (d) active personal participation in discussion and other group activities; (e) starting from powerlessness, thus, learning to regain control; (f) help giving and receiving, i.e., everybody relying upon other members' efforts, skills, knowledge, and concerns as its primary source of help; and (g) sharing common life experiences and problems.

In the 1980s, multiple-family group intervention was increasingly used among families of people with chronic and severe mental illness. Most of the clinical trials of family intervention for people with chronic and severe mental illness in the U.S. and U.K. were professional-led, didactic education programs, with patient participation, and focused on teaching family members how to take care of their patient at home and to prevent the patient's relapse (McFarlane, 2002). The use of mutual support groups as an approach to family intervention for these patients was not commonly accepted and used in Western countries until the late 1980s (Lefley, 1996). With increased attention and concerns about the health needs of family caregivers under the trend of family-based treatment for severe mental illness, many clinicians and researchers suggest that family intervention should not only contribute to patient recovery but also meet the families' psychosocial needs in caregiving (Solomon, 2000). Mutual support groups for family caregivers of a relative with severe mental illness—which provide information about mental illness, its treatment and community resources, opportunities to share feelings and experiences without fear of stigma, and emotional support and empathy—have been increasingly established throughout the U.S. One example is the National Alliance for the Mentally Ill in the early 1990s (Burland, 1998), purporting to meet the needs for social support and other aspects of mental health of these families.

Recent studies indicate significant positive effects of the use of mutual support groups for family-based treatment of patients with chronic mental health problems—such as eating disorders, dementia, and alcohol abuse—on some family-related outcomes (Colahan & Robinson, 2002; Doyle et al., 2003; McCallion & Toseland, 1995). Toseland and Rossiter (1989) reviewed 10 experimental or quasi-experimental studies of caregivers of patients with dementia in the 1980s and showed that a mutual support group can produce significant positive effects on families' psychosocial outcomes, such as burden and distress and coping with caregiving and social isolation, when compared with routine care. Colahan and Robinson (2002), in their study of family support groups conducted within an eating disorder service centre of a London NHS hospital, reported that family members are able to gain insight into their young relative's eating problem, improve family communication and, in presenting their experiences from the position of being in a similar predicament, provide support to participants in order to alleviate their sense of isolation and resistance to treatment. Despite the use of mutual support groups expanding into the domain of chronic mental illness, the positive values of this intervention for patients and their families are not conclusive (Heller et al., 1997).

While there are few clinical trials on mutual support group for families of patients with schizophrenia in Chinese and Western countries, the literature is replete with case studies, cross-sectional surveys, and qualitative and quasi-experimental approaches of a single treatment group, emphasizing the apparent benefits of the group in maintaining the psychological and social well-being of families (Ma, 1992; Heller et al., 1997). However, there is relatively little empirical evidence to support any enthusiastic claims of their benefits in improving families' functioning and satisfying their health needs (Pearson & Ning, 1997).

The paucity of empirical studies of mutual support groups for families of adult people with schizophrenia over the past two decades may be explained by the following factors. (a) The families tend to be socially isolated by the demands, burden and stigma of the illness, and their feeling of guilt and self blame for the illness; thus, they seldom seek help from professionals and other people outside the family (Cole & Reiss, 1993). (b) Support groups are an informal network of individuals depending on the leadership of peer volunteers, and challenges like maintaining momentum, ensuring regular evaluation and addressing individual and group changes are accentuated even more than in professional-led programs (Katz, 1997). (c) The goals, structure and activities of mutual support groups for these families vary as widely as the communities in which the groups are present; thus, it is difficult to replicate a standardized procedure of intervention and investigate its effectiveness and applicability in different settings and across cultures.

However, families caring for a relative with schizophrenia usually experience negative reactions from society towards patients and themselves, and many isolate themselves from their natural helping network due to feelings of shame and stigma. Mutual support tends to be viewed as a replacement support network for those in psychosocial crisis, one that, by its nature, is more appropriately able to provide empathy and support for participants who are "in the same boat" (Gidron, Guterman & Hartman, 1990). However, previous studies attempted to overcome some of the difficulties in design of a structured mutual support group program and tested its effectiveness in groups of families of people with schizophrenia in different developed countries.

All mutual support groups function as informal social support systems in that they promote an enduring pattern of continuous or intermittent ties that play a significant part in maintaining psychiatric and physical health over time. Social support theories broadly hold that social support and social networks are useful in promoting mental health because they (a) buffer the impact of stressful life events and (b) directly influence or reduce the occurrence of various mental disorders (Champion & Goodall, 1994; Lakey & Cohen, 2000). Studies demonstrate the influence of life events on the occurrence of various psychiatric and physical disorders, which appear to be mediated by adequate perceived social support (Champion, 1990; Chou et al., 1999). Cohen and Wills (1985), in their reviews of studies on families of mentally ill people, conclude that emotional and instrumental support from intimate social interactions can have a potential buffering effect on the impact of stressful events in caregiving.

Nevertheless, two of very few controlled trials conducted by Chien and Chan (2004) and Chien et al. (2006) amongst Chinese people in Hong Kong indicated that the mutual support group experienced significantly greater improvements in families' burden, functioning and number of support persons and length of patients' re-hospitalizations at 12- and 18-month follow-up. These findings provide preliminary evidence that mutual support groups can be an effective family-initiated, community-based intervention for Chinese people with schizophrenia.

# CONCLUSION

Despite the slow and patchy development of the use of pharmacological and psychosocial treatments in patients with schizophrenia, the dissemination of these interventions to patients is still the main approach within mental health services across Western and non-Western countries (Barbato & D'Avanzo, 2000). Families, particularly those family members who live with their relative with schizophrenia, often face and report a high level of psychological distress, social stigma, emotional frustration in the form of guilt and loneliness, and practical problems in living with and/or taking care of the patient at home. Several types of family-focused intervention, such as family psycho-education and behavioral family management programs, have been developed and found to be effective in meeting the needs of families in caring for a relative with schizophrenia. Recent reviews of clinical trials on family intervention in Western countries indicate that among these modes of family intervention the psycho-educational and supportive group programs are more effective in reducing patients' relapse and improving medication compliance up to one year's follow-up than the usual psychiatric care. However, there are important shortcomings in studies of family intervention, and limitations in our understanding of its effects for patients with schizophrenia and their families. These include the following:

a. Studies of the effects of these commonly-used modalities of family intervention on patient and family-related psychosocial outcomes, other than patient relapse and medication compliance, are inconclusive.
b. Implementation of family intervention techniques in routine practice has been hindered due mainly to inadequate staff training and supervision, scarce resources, or lack of availability of trained staff. Moreover, it may be difficult to maintain the efficacy of an intervention delivered over

many years compared to a relatively short-term intervention, which is subject to evaluation.

c. The great majority of family intervention studies in schizophrenia have been undertaken in Western developed countries. There have been only two studies in mainland China. Findings of Western studies cannot be easily generalized to non-Western populations because family interventions probably need to be adapted to meet cultural requirements if they are to be optimally effective
d. Little is known about the therapeutic components or mechanisms of these family psychosocial interventions, through which they produce their effects.

However, there is evidence that the psycho-education groups are effective in some chronic physical and mental illnesses. There is preliminary evidence from descriptive studies among people with schizophrenia in Western and non-Western cultures and, thus, this approach of family intervention should be empirically evaluated to establish its effectiveness in families of persons with schizophrenia.

Mutual support group programs require only limited training for nurses or other health professionals to serve as facilitators and provide a flexible, interactive, client-directed approach to help families cope with their caregiving role. Thus, the family support groups may be an effective alternative model of family intervention for schizophrenia. It is also important to test this intervention in Asian families who are part of a specific culture characterized by a strong sense of filial responsibility, close interdependence, and mutual support. Future study is recommended to build upon preliminary evidence of the effectiveness of mutual support groups for families dealing with schizophrenia in different countries and takes account, in its design, of the methodological limitations of previous studies of family intervention discussed in this chapter.

# REFERENCES


Anderson, C., Reiss, D., & Hogarty, G. (1986). *Schizophrenia and the family: a practitioner's guide to psycho-education and management.* New York: Guilford Press.

Anderson, J., & Adams, C. (1996). Family interventions in schizophrenia: An effective but underused treatment. *British Medical Journal,* 313 (7056), 505-506.

Arno, P. S., Levine, C., & Memmott, M. M. (1999). The economic value of informal caregiving. *Health Affairs,* 18, 182-188.

Asen, E. (2002). Multiple family therapy: An overview. *Journal of Family Therapy,* 24, 3-16.

Barbato, A., & D'Avanzo, B. (2000). Family interventions in schizophrenia and related disorders: A critical review of clinical trials. *Acta Psychiatrica Scandinavica,* 102 (2), 81-97.

Barnes, T. R. E., Hutton, S. B., Chapman, M. J., Mutsatsa, S., Puri, B. K., & Joyce, E. M. (2000). West London first episode study of schizophrenia: clinical correlates of duration of untreated psychosis. *British Journal of Psychiatry*, 177, 207-211.

Barrowclough, C., Haddock, G., Lowens, I., Connor, A., Pidliswyi, J., Tracey, N. (2001). Staff expressed emotion and causal attributions for client problems on a low security unit: An exploratory study. *Schizophrenia Bulletin,* 27 (3), 517-526.

Barrowclough, C., & Johnston, M. (1996). Distress, expressed emotion and attributions in relatives of schizophrenic patients. *Schizophrenia Bulletin,* 22 (4), .691-702.

Barrowclough, C., & Parle, M. (1997). Appraisal, psychological adjustment and expressed emotion in relatives of patients suffering from schizophrenia. *British Journal of Psychiatry,* 171 (1), 26-30.

Barrowclough, C., & Tarrier, N. (1992). *Families of schizophrenic patients: Cognitive behavioural intervention.* London: Chapman & Hall.

Bateson, D. H., Jackson, D., Haley, J., & Weakland, J. (1956). Towards a theory of schizophrenia. *Behavioral Science,* 1, .251-264.

Bebbington, P., & Kuipers, L. (1994). The predictive utility of expressed emotion in schizophrenia: an aggregate analysis. *Psychological Medicine,* 24 (3), 707-718.

Becker, T., Leese, M., Clarkson, P., Taylor, R. E., Turner, D., Kleckham, J., & Thornicroft, G. (1998). Links between social network and quality of life: An epidemiologically representative study of psychotic patients in south London. *Social Psychiatry & Psychiatric Epidemiology,* 33 (7), 229-304.

Bellack, A. S., Haas, G. L., Schooler, N. R., & Flory, J. D. (2000). Effects of behavioural family management on family communication and patient outcomes in schizophrenia. *British Journal of Psychiatry,* 177, 434-439.

Berglund, N., Vahlne, J. O., & Edman, A. (2003). Family intervention in schizophrenia: impact on family burden and attitude. *Social Psychiatry and Psychiatric Epidemiology,* 38 (3), 116-121.

Bernheim, K. F. (1987). Psychologists and families of the severely mentally ill: The role of family consultation. *American Psychologist,* 44 (3), 561-564.

Bernheim, K. F., & Lehman, A. F. (1985). *Working with families of the mentally ill.* New York: Norton.

Biegel, D. E., Robinson, E. A., & Kennedy, M. J. (2000). A review of empirical studies of interventions for families of persons with mental illness. *Research in Community and Mental Health,* 11, 97-130.

Bishop, P., Clilverd, A., Cooklin, A., & Hunt, U. (2002). Mental health matters: A multi-family framework for mental health intervention. *Journal of Family Therapy,* 24, 31-45.

Brooker, C. (2001). Decade of evidence-based training for work with people with serious mental health problems: Progress in the development of psychosocial interventions. *Journal of Mental Health,* 10, 17-31.

Brown, G. W., Monick, E. M., Carstairs, G. M., & Wing, J. K. (1962). Influence of family life on the course of schizophrenia illness. *British Journal of Preventive Social Medicine,* 16, 55-68.

Brown, G. W., Birley, J. L. T., & Wing, J. K. (1972). Influence of family life on the course of schizophrenic disorder. *British Journal of Psychiatry,* 121, 241-258.

Brennan, G. (2000). Stress vulnerability model of serious mental illness. In: C. Gamble, & G. Brennan (Eds.), *Working with Serious Mental Illness: A Manual for Clinical Practice* (pp. 29-40). Edinburgh: Harcourt Publishers Ltd.

Budd, R. J., Oles, G., & Hughes, I. C. T. (1998). The relationship between coping style and burden in the carers of relatives with schizophrenia. *Acta Psychiatrica Scandinavica,* 98, 304-309.

Burland, J. (1998). Family-to-family: A trauma-and-recovery model of family education. In: Lefley, H. (Ed.*), Family Coping with Mental Illness: The Cultural Context* (pp. 33-41). San Francisco, CA: Jossey-Boss Publishers:

Bustillo, J. R., Lauriello, J., Horan, W. P., & Keith, S. J. (2001). The psychosocial treatment of schizophrenia: An update. *American Journal of Psychiatry*, 158 (2), 163-175.

Butzlaff, R. L., & Hooley, J. M. (1998). Expressed emotion and psychiatric relapse: A meta-analysis. *Archives of General Psychiatry,* 55 (6), 547-552.

Canive, J. M., Sanz-Fuentenebro, J., Vazquez, C., Qualls, C., Fuentenebro, F., Perez, I. G., & Tuason, V.B. (1996). Family psychoeducational support groups in Spain: Parents' distress and burden at nine-month follow-up. *Annuals of Clinical Psychiatry*, 8 (2), 71-79.

Champion, L. A. (1990). The relationship between social vulnerability and the occurrence of severely threatening life events. *Psychological Medicine*, 20 (suppl 1), 157-161.

Champion, L. A., & Goodall, G. M. (1994). Social support and mental health: positive and negative aspects. In: D. Tantam, & M. J. Birchwood (Eds.), *Seminars in Psychology and the Social Sciences* (pp. 238-259). London: Royal College of Psychiatrists.

Chan, S. & Yu, I. W. (2004). Quality of life of clients with schizophrenia. *Journal of Advanced Nursing,* 45, 72-83.

Chien, W. T., & Chan, C. W. S. (2004). One-year follow-up of a multiple-family group intervention for Chinese families of patients with schizophrenia. *Psychiatric Services, 55* (11), 1276-1284.

Chien, W. T., Chan, S., Morrissey, J., & Thompson, D. (2005). Effectiveness of a mutual support group for families of patients with schizophrenia. *Journal of Advanced Nursing,* 51 (6), 595-608.

Chien, W. T., Chan, W. C. S., & Thompson, D. R. (2006). Effects of a mutual support group for families of Chinese people with schizophrenia: 18-month follow-up. *British Journal of Psychiatry, 189*, 41-49.

Chien, W. T., & Norman, I. (2004). The validity and reliability of a Chinese version of the Family Burden Interview Schedule. *Nursing Research,* 53 (5), 314-322.

Chou, K. R. (2000). Caregiver burden: A concept analysis. *Journal of Pediatric Nursing,* 15 (6), 398-407.

Chou, K. R., LaMontagne, L. L., & Hepworth, J. T. (1999). Burden experienced by caregivers of relatives with dementia in Taiwan. *Nursing Research*, 48 (4), 206-214.

Chou, K. R., Liu, S. Y., & Chu, H. (2002). The effects of support groups on caregivers of patients with schizophrenia. *International Journal of Nursing Studies,* 39 (7), 713-722.

Clausen, J. A., & Yarrow, M. R. (Eds.) (1955). The impact of mental illness on the family. *Journal of Social Issues,* 11, 3-64.

Cohen, S., & Wills, T. A. (1985). Stress, social support and the buffering hypothesis. *Psychological Bulletin,* 98 (2), 310-357.

Colahan, M., & Robinson, P. H. (2002). Multi-family groups in the treatment of young adults with eating disorders. *Journal of Family Therapy,* 24, 17-30.

Cole, R. E., & Reiss, D. (Eds.) (1993). *How Do Families Cope with Chronic Illness?* Hillsdale: NJ, Lawrence Erlbaum Associates, Inc.

Cook, J. A., Heller, T., & Pickett-Schenk, S. A. (1999). The effects of support group participation on caregiver burden among parents of adult offspring with severe mental illness. *Family Relations,* 48 (4), 405-410.

Cook, J. A., Lefley, H. P., Pickett, S. A., & Cohler, B. J. (1994). Age and family burden among parents of offspring with severe mental illness. *American Journal of Orthopsychiatry,* 64, 435-447.

Cook, J. A., & Wright, E. R. (1995). Medical sociology and the study of severe mental illness: Reflections on past accomplishments and directions for future research. *Journal of Health and Social Behaviour,* 36 (Extra issue), 95-114.

Cuijpers, P. (1999). The effects of family interventions on relatives' burden: A meta-analysis. *Journal of Mental Health,* 8 (3), 275-285.

Dare, C., & Eisler, I. (2000). A multi-family group day treatment for adolescent eating disorder. *European Eating Disorders Review,* 8, 4–18.

Department of Health, UK (1999) *National Service Framework for Mental health: Modern Standards & Services Models*. London: NHS, Department of Health.

Dixon, L., Adams, C., & Luckstead, A. (2000). Update on family psycho-education for schizophrenia. *Schizophrenia Bulletin,* 26 (1), 5-20.

Dixon, L., Lyles, A., Scott, J., Postrado, L., Goldman, H., & McGlynn, E. (1999). Services to families of adults with schizophrenia: From treatment recommendations to dissemination. *Psychiatric Services,* 50 (2), 233-238.

Doyle, M., Carr, A., Rowen, S., Galvin, P., Lyons, S., & Cooney, G. (2003). Family-oriented treatment for people with alcohol problems in Ireland: A comparison of the effectiveness of residential and community-based programmes. *Journal of Family Therapy,* 25, 15-40.

Drake, R. J., Haley, C. J., Akhar, S., & Lewis, S. (2000). Causes and consequences of duration of untreated psychosis in schizophrenia. *British Journal of Psychiatry,* 177 (6), 511-515.

Dunkin, J. J., & Hanley, C.A. (1998). Dementia caregiver burden: A review of the literature and guidelines for assessment and intervention. *American Academy of Neurology,* 51 (Suppl 1), S53-S60.

Dyck, D. G., Hendryx, M. S., Short, R. A., Voss, W. D., & McFarlane, W. R. (2002). Service use among patients with schizophrenia in psycho-educational multiple-family group treatment. *Psychiatric Services,* 53 (6), 749-754.

Fadden, G. (1998). Research update: Psychoeducational family interventions. *Journal of Family Therapy,* 20, 293-309.

Fadden, G. (2001). Family intervention. In: C. Brooker, & J. Repper (Eds.), *Serious Mental Problems in the Community: Policy, Practice and Research* (pp. 159-183). Edinburgh: Balliere-Tindall.

Falloon, I. R. H., Boyd, J. L., & McGill, C. W. (1984). *Family care of schizophrenia.* New York: Guilford Press.

Falloon, I. R. H., Boyd, J. L., McGill, C. W., Razani, J., Moss, H. B., & Gilderman, A. M. (1982). Family management in the prevention of exacerbations of schizophrenia: a controlled study. *New England Journal of Medicine,* 306 (4), 1437-1440.

Falloon, I. R. H., & Liberman, R. P. (1983). Interactions between drug and psychosocial therapy in schizophrenia. *Schizophrenia Bulletin*, 9, 543-554.

Falloon, I. R. H., Liberman, R. P., Lillie, F. J., Vaughan, K. (1981). Family therapy of schizophrenics with high risk of relapse. *Family Process*, 20, 211-221.

Falloon, I. R. H., Boyd, J. L., McGill, C. W., Williamson, M., Razani, J., Moss, H. B., Gilderman, A. M., & Simpson, G. M. (1985). Family management in the prevention of morbidity in schizophrenia. Clinical outcome of a two-year longitudinal study. *Archives of General Psychiatry,* 42 (9), 887-896.

Flanagan, D. A. J., & Wagner, H. L. (1991). Expressed emotion and panic-fear in the prediction of diet treatment compliance. *British Journal of Clinical Psychology,* 30 (3), 231-240.

Gerlsma, C., & Hale III, W. W. (1997). Predictive power and construct validity of the Level of Expressed Emotion scale. *British Journal of Psychiatry,* 170, 520-525.

Gidron, B., Guterman, N. B., & Hartman, H. (1990). Stress and coping patterns of participants and non-participants in self-help groups for parents of the mentally ill. *Community Mental Health Journal,* 26 (6), 483-496.

Greenberg, J. S., Greenley, J. R., & Benedict, P. (1994). Contributions of persons with serious mental illness to their families. *Hospital and Community Psychiatry,* 45, 475-480.

Hatfield, A. B. (Ed.) (1994). Family interventions in mental illness. *New Directions for Mental Health Services,* No. 62. San Francisco, CA: Jossey-Bass Inc.

Hatfield, A. B., & Lefley, H. P. (1987). Families of the mentally ill: *Coping and adaptation.* New York: Guilford Press.

Hazel, N. A., McDonell, M. G., Short, R. A., Berry, C. M., Voss, W. D., Rodgers, M. L., & Dyck, D. G. (2004). Impact of multiple-family groups for outpatients with schizophrenia on caregivers' distress and resources. *Psychiatric Services,* 55, 35-41.

Heller, T., Roccoforte, J. A., & Cook, J. A. (1997). Predictors of support group participation among families of persons with mental illness. *Family Relations,* 46 (4), 437-442.

Hirsch, S., & Leff, J. (1975). *Abnormalities in parents of schizophrenics.* Maudsley Monograph No. 22. London: Oxford University Press.

Hogarty, G. E., Anderson, C. M., Reiss, D. J., Kornblith, S. J., Greenwald, D. P., Ulrich, R. F., & Carter, M. (1991). Family psychoeducation, social skills training, and maintenance chemotherapy in the aftercare treatment of schizophrenia, II: Two-year effects of a controlled study on relapse and adjustment. *Archives of General Psychiatry,* 48 (5), 340-347.

Hogarty, G. E., Kornblith, S. J., Greenwald, D., DiBarry, A. L., Cooley, S., Ulrich, R. F., Carter, M., & Flesher, S. (1997). Three-year trials of personal therapy among schizophrenic patients living with or independent of family I. Description of study and effects on relapse rates. *American Journal of Psychiatry,* 154 (11), 1504-1513.

Iodice, J. D., & Wodarski, J. S. (1987). Aftercare treatment for schizophrenics living at home. *Social Work*, 32 (2), 122-128.

Ivanović, M., Vuletić, Z., & Bebbington, P. (1994). Expressed emotion in the families of patients with schizophrenia and its influence on the course of illness. *Social Psychiatry and Psychiatric Epidemiology,* 29, 61-65.

Karanci, A. N., & Inandilar, H. (2002). Predictors of components of expressed emotion in major caregivers of Turkish patients with schizophrenia. *Social Psychiatry and Psychiatric Epidemiology,* 37, 80-88.

Katz, L. F. (1997). *Self-help and Support Groups: A Handbook for Practitioners. Thousand Oaks,* CA: Sage Publications.

Kavanagh, D. J., Piatkowska, O., Clarke, D., O'Halloran, P., Manicavasagar, V., Rosen, A., & Tennant, C. (1993) Application of cognitive-behavioural family intervention for schizophrenia in multi-disciplinary teams: What can the matter be? *Australian Psychologist,* 28, 181-188.

Kavanagh, S., Opit, L., Knapp, M., & Beecham, J. (1995). Schizophrenia: Shifting the balance of care. *Social Psychiatry and Psychiatric Epidemiology,* 30 (5), 206-212.

Koettgen, C., Soennichsen, I., Mollenhauer, K., & Jurth, R. (1984). Group therapy with the families of schizophrenic patients: Results of the Hamburg Camberwell Family Interview study III. *International Journal of Family Psychiatry,* 5 (1), 83-94.

Kuipers, E., Leff, J., & Lam, D. (2002). *Family Work for Schizophrenia* (2nd ed.). London: The Royal College of Psychiatrists.

Lakey, B. & Cohen, S. (2000). Support theory and measurement. In: S. Cohen, L. Underwood, & B. Gottlieb, (Eds), *Measuring and intervening in social support* (pp. 29-52). New York: Oxford University press.

Leff, J. (1994). Working with the families of schizophrenic patients. *British Journal of Psychiatry,* 164 (1), 71-76.

Leff, J., Berkowitz, R., Shavit, N., Strachen, A., Glass, I., & Vaughn, C. (1989). A trial of family therapy vs a relative group for schizophrenia. *British Journal of Psychiatry,* 154 (1), 58-66.

Leff, J., Berkowitz, R., Shavit, N., Strachen, A., Glass, I., & Vaughn, C. (1990). A trial of family therapy vs a relatives' group for schizophrenia: Two-year follow-up. *British Journal of Psychiatry,* 157 (4), 571-577.

Lefley, H. P. (1996). Family Caregiving in Mental Illness. *Thousand Oaks,* CA: Sage Publications.

Leff, J., & Vaughn, C. (1985). *Expressed Emotion in Families.* New York: Guilford.

Lehman, A. F., & Steinwachs, D. M. (1998). At issue - Translating research into practice: the Schizophrenia Patient Outcomes Research Team (PORT) treatment recommendations. *Schizophrenia Bulletin,* 24 (1), 1–9.

Lehman, A. F., Steinwachs, D. M., & the Survey Co-investigators of the PORT project (1998) Patterns of usual care for schizophrenia: Initial results from the schizophrenia patient outcomes research team (PORT) client survey. *Schizophrenia Bulletin,* 24 (1), 11-20.

Lemmens, G. M., Wauters, S., Heireman, M., Eisler, I., Lietaer, G., & Sabbe, B. (2003). Beneficial factors in family discussion groups of a psychiatric day clinic: Perceptions by the therapeutic team and the families of the therapeutic process. *Journal of Family Therapy,* 25, 41-63.

Levene, J. E., Newman, F., & Jeffries, J. J. (1989). Focal family therapy outcome study, I: Patient and family functioning. *Canadian Journal of Psychiatry,* 34 (7), 641-647.

Linszen, D., Dingemans, P., Van der Does, J. W., Nugter, A., Scholte, P., Lenior, R., & Goldstein, M. J. (1996). Treatment, expressed emotion and relapse in recent onset schizophrenic disorders. *Psychological Medicine,* 26 (2), 333-342.

Loukissa, D. A. (1995). Family burden in chronic mental illness: A review of research studies. *Journal of Advanced Nursing,* 21 (2), 248-255.

Lukens, E., Thorning, H., & Herman, D. (1999). Family psychoeducation in schizophrenia: Emerging themes and challenges. *Journal of Practice in Psychological and Behavioural Health,* November, 314-325.

Ma, J. (1992). Social support, mutual aid groups, the mentally ill and their families. *Hong Kong Journal of Mental Health,* 21 (1), 16-27.

Ma, K. Y., & Yip, K. S. (1997). The importance of an effective psychiatric community care service for chronic mental patients in Hong Kong. *Hong Kong Journal of Mental Health,* 26 (1), 28-35.

Mari, J. J., & Streiner, D. (1996). Family intervention for people with schizophrenia. In: *The Cochrane Library*, Issue 1, 1996. Oxford: Cochrane Library Update Software [Electronic database].

Marsh, D. T. (1994). The psychodynamic model and services for families: Issues and strategies. In: H. Lefley, & M. Wasow (Eds.), *Helping Families Cope with Mental Illness* (pp.105-128). Chur, Switzerland: Harwood Academic Publishers.

Marsh, D. T. (1998). Serious Mental Illness and the Family: *The Practitioner's Guide.* New York: John Wiley & Sons.

Marsh, D., & Johnson, D. (1997). The family experience of mental illness: Implications for interventions. *Professional Psychological Research and Practice,* 28, 229-237.

Martens, L., & Addington, J. (2001). The psychological well being of family members of individuals with schizophrenia. *Social Psychiatry and Psychiatric Epidemiology*, 36, 128-133.

Maurin, J. T., & Boyd, C. B. (1990). Burden of mental illness on the family: A critical review. *Archives of Psychiatric Nursing,* 4 (2),.99-107.

McCallion, P., & Toseland, R. W. (1995). Supportive group interventions with caregivers of frail older adults. *Social Work with Groups,* 18 (1), 11-25.

McDonell, M. G., Short, R. A., Berry, C. M., & Dyck, D. G. (2004). Burden in schizophrenia caregivers: *Impact of family psychoeducation and awareness of patient suicidality. Family Process,* 42 (1), 91-103.

McFarlane, W. R. (1994). Multiple family groups and psycho-education in the treatment of schizophrenia. *New Directions for Mental Health Services,* 62, 13-22.

McFarlane, W. R. (2002). *Multifamily groups in the treatment of severe psychiatric disorders.* New York: Guilford Press.

McFarlane, W. R., Dixon, L., Lukens, E., & Lucksted, A. (2003). Family psychoeducation and schizophrenia: A review of the literature. *Journal of Marital & Family Therapy,* 29 (2), 223-245.

McFarlane, W. R., Link, B., Dushay, R., Marchal, J., & Crilly, J. (1995). Psychoeducational multiple family groups: Four-year relapse outcome in schizophrenia. *Family Process,* 34 (2), 127-144.

McFarlane, W. R., Stastny, P., & Deakins, S. (1992). Family aided assertive community treatment: A comprehensive rehabilitation and intensive case management approach for persons with schizophrenic disorders. *New Directions in Mental Health Services,* 53, 43-54.

Meredith, W. H., Abbott, D. A., Tsai, R., Zheng, F. M., & Meredith, W. H. (1994). Healthy family functioning in Chinese cultures: An exploratory study using the Circumplex Model. *International Journal of the Sociology of the Family,* 24 (1), 147-157.

Montero, I., Asencio, A., Hernandez, I., Masanet, M .J., Lacruz, M., Bellver, F., Iborra, M., & Ruiz, I. (2001). Two strategies for family intervention in schizophrenia: *A randomised trial in a Mediterranean environment. Schizophrenia Bulletin,* 27 (6), 661-670.

Mueser, K. T. (2003). *Mental Health Guidelines - Family services for severe mental illness.* February 2003. Illinois, US: Behavioral Health Recovery Management, Fayette Companies & Chestnut Health Systems.

Mueser, K. T., & Gingerich, S. (1994*). Coping with Schizophrenia: A Guide for Families*. Oakland, CA: New Harbinger Publications.

Mueser, K. T., & Glynn, S. M. (1999). *Behavioral family therapy for psychiatric disorders,* 2nd edn. Oakland, CA: New Harbinger Publications.

National Collaborating Centre for Mental Health. (2002). *Clinical Guideline 1 - Schizophrenia: Core interventions in the treatment and management of schizophrenia in primary and secondary care.* December 2002. London: National Institute for Clinical Excellence.

National Health Service Centre for Reviews and Dissemination. (2001). *Undertaking systematic reviews of research on effectiveness: CRD's guidance for those carrying out or commissioning reviews* (CRD Report Number 4, 2nd edn.). York, UK: University of York.

Noh, S., & Turner, R. J. (1987). Living with psychiatric patients: Implications for the mental health and family members. *Social Science and Medicine,* 25 (3), 263-272.

Nolan, M., Lundh, U., Grant, G., & Keady, J. (Eds.) (2003). *Partnerships in Family Care: Understanding the Caregiving Career.* Maidenhead, U.K.: Open University Press.

Ohaeri, J. U. (2003). The burden of caregiving in families with a mental illness: A review of 2002. *Current Opinion in Psychiatry,* 16 (4), 457-465.

Pearson, V., & Ning, S. P. (1997). Family care in schizophrenia: An undervalued resource. In: C. L. W. Chan, & N. Rhind (Eds.), *Social Work Intervention in Health Care. The Hong Kong Scene* (pp. 317-336.). Hong Kong: Hong Kong University Press.

Penn, D. L., & Mueser, K. T. (1996). Research update on the psychosocial treatment of schizophrenia. *American Journal of Psychiatry*, 153 (5), 607-617.

Pharoah, F. M., Mari, J. J., & Streiner, D. (2001). *Family intervention for schizophrenia.* The Cochrane Library Reviews, Issue 3, 2001. Oxford: Cochrane Library Update Software [Electronic database].

Pilling, S., Bebbington, P., Kuipers, E., Garety, P., Geddes, J., Orbach, G., & Morgan, C. (2002). Psychological treatments in schizophrenia, I: Meta-analysis of family intervention and cognitive behaviour therapy. *Psychological Medicine,* 32, 763-782.

Posner, C. M., Wilson, K. G., Kral, M. J., Lander, S., & McIlwraith, R. D. (1992). Family psychoeducational support groups in schizophrenia. *American Journal of Orthopsychiatry,* 62 (2), 206-218.

Raune, D., Kuipers, E., Bebbington, P. E. (2004). Expressed emotion at first-episode psychosis: Investigating a carer appraisal model. *British Journal of Psychiatry,* 184, 321-326.

Reinhard, C. S. (1994). Living with mental illness: Effects of professional support and personal control on caregiver burden. *Research in Nursing and Health*, 17, 79-88.

Repper, J., & Brooker, C. (1998). Serious mental health problems in the community: The significance of policy, practice and research. In: C. Brooker, & J. Repper (Eds.), *Serious Mental Health Problems in the Community: Policy, Practice and Research* (pp. 8-30). London: Bailliere-Tindall.

Rose, L., Mallinson, R. K., & Walton-Moss, B. (2002). A grounded theory of families responding to mental illness. *Western Journal of Nursing Studies,* 24, 16-36.

Rungreangkulkij, S., & Gilliss, C. L. (2000). Conceptual approaches to studying family caregiving for persons with severe mental illness. *Journal of Family Nursing,* 6 (4), 341-366.

Saunders, J. C. (1999). Family functioning in families providing care for a family member with schizophrenia. *Issues in Mental Health Nursing,* 20 (2), 95-113.

Scazufca, M., & Kuipers, E. (1999). Coping strategies in relatives of people with schizophrenia before and after psychiatric admission. *British Journal of Psychiatry,* 174 (2), 154-158.

Schene, A. H. (1990). Objective and subjective dimensions of family burden. Toward an integrative framework for research. *Social Psychiatry and Psychiatric Epidemiology,* 25, 289-297.

Schene, A. H., Tessler, R. C., & Gamanche, G. M. (1994). Instruments measuring family or caregiver burden in severe mental illness. *Social Psychiatry and Psychiatric Epidemiology,* 29, 228-240.

Schooler, N. R., Keith, S. J., Severe, J. B., Matthews, S. M., Bellack, A. S., Glick, I. D., et al. (1997). Relapse and re-hospitalization during the maintenance treatment of schizophrenia. *The effects of dose reduction and family treatment. Archives of General Psychiatry,* 54 (5), 453-463.

Schultz, R., & Beach, S.R. (1999). Caregiving as a risk factor for mortality: The caregiver health effects study. *JAMA,* 282 (23), 2215-2219.

Schultz, R., & Sherwood, P.R. (2008). Physical and mental health effects of family caregiving. *American Journal of Nursing,* 108 (Suppl. 9), 23-27.

Sellwood, W., Barrowclough, C., Tarrier, N., Quinn, J., Mainwaring, J., & Lewis, S. (2001). Needs-based cognitive-behavioural family intervention for carers of patients suffering from schizophrenia: 12-month follow-up. *Acta Psychiatrica Scandinavica,* 104 (5), 346-355.

Sidley, G. L., Smith, J., & Howells, K. (1991). Is it ever too late to learn? Information provision to relatives of long-term schizophrenia sufferers. *Behavioural Psychotherapy*, 19, 496-500.

Solomon, P. (2000). Interventions for families of individuals with schizophrenia: Maximising outcomes for their relatives. *Disease Management and Health Outcomes,* 8 (4), .211-221.

Solomon, P., & Draine, J. (1995). Subjective burden among family members of mentally ill adults: Relation to stress, coping, and adaptation. *American Journal of Orthopsychiatry,* 65, 419-427.

Solomon, P., Draine, J., Mannion, E., & Meisel, M. (1996). The impact of individualised consultation and group workshop of family education interventions on ill relative outcomes. *Journal of Nervous and Mental Diseases,* 184 (4), 252-254.

Spiegel, D., Bloom, J. R,. Kraemer, H. C., & Gottheil, E. (1989). Effect of psychosocial treatment on survival of patients with metastatic breast cancer. *Lancet,* 2 (8668), 888-891.

Stein, L. I., & Santos, A. B. (1998). *Assertive community treatment of persons with severe mental illness.* New York: Norton.

Steinglass, P. (1998). Multiple family discussion groups for patients with chronic medical illness. *Families, Systems and Health, 16*, 55-70.

Tarrier, N. (1991). Some aspects of family interventions in schizophrenia: I. Adherence to intervention programmes. *British Journal of Psychiatry*, 159 (4), 475-480.

Tarrier, N., Barrowclough, C., Porceddu, K., & Fitzpatrick, E. (1994). The Salford Family Intervention Project for schizophrenic relapse prevention: Five and eight-year accumulating relapses. *British Journal of Psychiatry,* 165 (6), 829-832.

Tarrier, N., Barrowclough, C., Vaughn, C., Bamrah, J., Porceddu, K., Watts, S., & Freeman, H. (1989). Community management of schizophrenia: A two year follow-up of a behavioural intervention with families. *British Journal of Psychiatry,* 154 (5), 625-628.

Telles, C., Karno, M., Mintz, J., Paz, G., Arias, M., Tucker, D., & Lopez, S. (1995). Immigrant families coping with schizophrenia. Behavioural family intervention vs. case management with a low-income Spanish-speaking population. *British Journal of Psychiatry,* 167 (4), 473-479.

Thornicroft, G., & Susser, E. (2001). Evidence-based psychotherapeutic interventions in the community care of schizophrenia. *British Journal of Psychiatry,* 178 (1), 2-4.

Toseland, R. W., & Rossiter, C. M. (1989). Group interventions to support family caregivers: A review and analysis. *Gerontologist,* 29 (4), 438-448.

Ustun, T. B. (1999). The global burden of mental disorders. *American Journal of Public Health,* 89, 1315-1318.

Vaughan, K., Doyle, M., McConaghy, N., Blaszczynski, A., Fox, A., & Tarrier, N. (1992). The Sydney Intervention Trial: A controlled trial of relatives' counselling to reduce schizophrenic relapse. *Social Psychiatry and Psychiatric Epidemiology,* 27 (1), 16-21.

Vaughn, C. E., & Leff, J. P. (1976). The measurement of expressed emotion in the families of psychiatric patients. *British Journal of Social and Clinical Psychology,* 15, 157-165.

Vitaliano, P. P., Zhang, J., & Scanlan, J. M. (2003). Is caregiving hazardous to one's physical health? A meta-analysis. *Psychological Bulletin*, 129 (6), 946-972.

Wearden, A. J., Tarrier, N., Barrowclough, C., Zastowny, T. R., Rahill, A. A. (2000). A review of expressed emotion research in health care. *Clinical Psychology Review,* 20(5), 633-636.

Woods, N. F., Haberman, M. R., & Packard, N. J. (1993). Demands of illness and individual, dyadic and family adaptation in chronic illness. *Western Journal of Nursing Research,* 15 (1), 15-30.

World Health Organization. (2007). World Health Statistics 2007. Geneva: WHO.

Xiong, W., Philips, M. R., Hu, X., Wang, R., Dai, Q., Kleinman, J., & Kleinman, A. (1994). Family-based intervention for schizophrenic patients in China. A randomised controlled trial. *British Journal of Psychiatry,* 165 (3), 239-247.

Zastowny, T. R., Lehman, A. F., Cole, R. E., & Kane, C. (1992). Family management of schizophrenia: A comparison of behavioural and supportive family treatment. Psychiatric *Quarterly,* 63 (2), 159-186.

Zhang, M., Wang, M., Li, J., & Philips, M. R. (1994). A randomized controlled trial of family intervention for 78 first-episode male schizophrenic patients: An 18-month study in Suzhou, Jiangsu. *British Journal of Psychiatry,* 165 (Suppl 24), 96-102.

Zola, I. K. (1991). Bringing our bodies and ourselves back in: Reflections on a past, present, and future 'Medical Sociology'. *Journal of Health and Social Behaviour,* 32 (1), 1-16.

# INDEX

## D



## E

## F



## G



## H



## I

## J



## L



## M



## N



## O



## P

## Q



## R



## S

## T



## V

## W



## Y